Small Animal
**Medical
Differential
Diagnosis**

A BOOK OF LISTS

SECOND EDITION

Small Animal
Medical
Differential
Diagnosis

A BOOK OF LISTS

Mark S. Thompson

Diplomate, American Board of Veterinary Practitioners
Certified in Canine/Feline Practice
Brevard Animal Hospital
Brevard, North Carolina

ELSEVIER

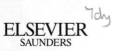

SIH
636.0896075 THD
7dy

ELSEVIER
SAUNDERS

3251 Riverport Lane
St. Louis, Missouri 63043

SMALL ANIMAL MEDICAL DIFFERENTIAL DIAGNOSIS:
A BOOK OF LISTS, SECOND EDITION   ISBN: 978-1-4557-4454-1

Notices

Knowledge and best practice in this field are constantly changing. As new research and experience
broaden our understanding, changes in research methods, professional practices, or medical
treatment may become necessary.

Practitioners and researchers must always rely on their own experience and knowledge in
evaluating and using any information, methods, compounds, or experiments described herein.
In using such information or methods they should be mindful of their own safety and the safety
of others, including parties for whom they have a professional responsibility.

With respect to any drug or pharmaceutical products identified, readers are advised to check
the most current information provided (i) on procedures featured or (ii) by the manufacturer
of each product to be administered, to verify the recommended dose or formula, the method
and duration of administration, and contraindications. It is the responsibility of practitioners,
relying on their own experience and knowledge of their patients, to make diagnoses, to
determine dosages and the best treatment for each individual patient, and to take all appropriate
safety precautions.

To the fullest extent of the law, neither the Publisher nor the authors, contributors, or editors,
assume any liability for any injury and/or damage to persons or property as a matter of products
liability, negligence or otherwise, or from any use or operation of any methods, products,
instructions, or ideas contained in the material herein.

Library of Congress Cataloging-in-Publication Data

Thompson, Mark S., author.
  Small animal medical differential diagnosis : a book of lists / Mark S. Thompson. – Second edition.
    p. ; cm.
  Includes index.
  ISBN 978-1-4557-4454-1 (pbk.)
  I. Title.
  [DNLM: 1. Dog Diseases–diagnosis–Handbooks. 2. Cat Diseases–diagnosis–Handbooks. 3. Diagnosis,
  Differential–Handbooks. SF 991]
  636.089'6075–dc23

                                                                        2013008764

Content Strategy Director: Penny S Rudolph
Associate Content Developer: Katie Starke
Publishing Services Manager: Catherine Albright Jackson
Senior Project Manager: Mary Pohlman
Project Manager: Anitha Sivaraj
Book Designer: Jessica Williams

Printed in the United States of America

Last digit is the print number: 9 8 7 6 5 4 3 2 1

Working together
to grow libraries in
developing countries

www.elsevier.com • www.bookaid.org

To my wife Sandi for 30 years of marriage.

When I was asked by Elsevier to create a second edition of *Small Animal Differential Diagnosis: A Book of Lists*, I envisioned an easy process of updating the lists of the first edition and adding some new material. I couldn't have been more wrong. The goal was to duplicate the format of the first edition: a quick, concise, and practical reference to differential diagnosis, etiology, laboratory values, and classification of clinical signs and medical disorders in dogs and cats. As I reviewed each list I was surprised to see how many needed to be revised. In fact, nearly all of the lists required additions, subtractions, or sometimes complete reorganization. A project like this one is a great illustration of how much the veterinary medical literature expands in a 6-year period. Once again, this text will be a pocket-sized, rapid reference or an electronic application. Its greatest value will be to aid the clinician in making reliable on-the-scene decisions and to allow veterinary students and interns to more fully participate in clinical rounds with their instructors. It will also be used by the more seasoned practitioner to come up with those more esoteric differentials that we sometimes forget to include in our list of potential diagnoses.

The lists in this book have been compiled from comprehensive veterinary references published by Elsevier, especially:

- Ettinger and Feldman: *Textbook of Veterinary Internal Medicine,* seventh edition and
- Nelson and Couto: *Small Animal Internal Medicine,* fourth edition.

Also consulted for information were:

- Henry and Higginbotham: *Cancer Management in Small Animal Practice*
- Beaver: *Canine Behavior: Insights and Answers,* second edition
- Landsberg: *Handbook of Behavior Problems of the Dog and Cat,* second edition
- Bonagura: *Kirk's Current Veterinary Therapy XIV*
- Maggs et al: *Slatter's Fundamentals of Veterinary Ophthalmology,* fifth edition
- Willard and Tvedten: *Small Animal Clinical Diagnosis by Laboratory Methods,* fifth edition
- Fossum: *Small Animal Surgery,* fourth edition

The reader is encouraged to consult these and other texts for more detailed information.

About the Book

As with the first edition, the lists are divided into three parts and serve as a concise guide to the differential diagnosis, etiology, laboratory abnormalities, and classification of clinical signs and medical disorders in dogs and cats. Part One contains lists based on clinical signs that may be identified by the clinician. Part Two approaches differential diagnosis from a systems perspective. Fifteen body systems are represented. Part Three once again is a quick reference of laboratory tests and gives typical normal ranges and differential diagnoses based on test results. Overall the book comprises 400 lists, 60 of which are new to this edition. In all lists an attempt has been made to prioritize them from least common to most common.

Acknowledgments

I wish to thank my fellow veterinarians at Brevard Animal Hospital: Dr. Christine Weaver, Dr. Clyde Brooks, Dr. Chad Lothamer, and Dr. Alana Terrell. They were a sounding board for ideas and helped me discover deficiencies in the first edition. In addition, our discussions about cases helped me determine new lists that needed to be generated.

CONTENTS

PART TWO
Systemic Approach to Differential Diagnosis, *77*

Small Animal
**Medical
Differential
Diagnosis**

PART ONE

Clinical Signs Approach to Differential Diagnosis

Abdominal Distension

Organomegaly

Hepatomegaly (infiltrative, inflammatory, lipidosis, neoplasia)
Splenomegaly (infiltrative, inflammatory, neoplasia, hematoma)
Renomegaly (neoplasia, infiltrative)
Miscellaneous neoplasia (GI tract, ovaries, uterus, pancreas, prostate, adrenal glands)
Generalized neoplasia (carcinomatosis, lymphosarcoma)
Granuloma (pythiosis, aspergillosis)
Pregnancy

Fluid

Contained in Organs

Congestion resulting from splenic torsion or volvulus, or hepatic congestion from right-sided heart failure
Cysts (paraprostatic, perinephric, hepatic)
Hydronephrosis
Distended urinary bladder
Obstruction of intestines or stomach
Ileus
Pyometra

Free Fluid in Abdomen

Transudate (portal hypertension, right-sided heart failure, hypoproteinemia secondary to protein-losing enteropathy, protein-losing nephropathy, or hepatic failure)
Modified transudate (neoplasia, postsinusoidal portal hypertension, right-sided heart failure, heartworm caval syndrome, liver disease)
Exudate (pancreatitis, feline infectious peritonitis, urine, bile, neoplasia, bowel perforation, foreign body)
Chyle (trauma, neoplasia, infection, right-sided heart failure)
Blood (coagulopathy, trauma, neoplasia)

Gas

Contained in Organs

Gastric dilatation/volvulus
Intestines secondary to obstruction
Parenchymal organs infected with gas-producing bacteria

Free in Abdomen

Iatrogenic (after laparoscopy, laparotomy)
Rupture of gastrointestinal tract or uterus

Fat

Obesity/lipoma

Weakened Abdominal Musculature

Hyperadrenocorticism

Feces

Obstipation/megacolon

Abdominal Effusions and Ascites

Transudate (<1000 Cells, <2.5 Total Solids, <1.017 Specific Gravity)

Portal Hypertension
Presinusoidal or sinusoidal liver disease
Right-sided heart failure

Hypoalbuminemia (see Albumin p. 286)
Liver failure
Protein-losing enteropathy

Glomerulopathy

Modified Transudate (>1000 but <10000 Cells, 2.5-5.0 Total Solids, <1.025 Specific Gravity)

Postsinusoidal Portal Hypertension

Right-Sided Heart Failure
Heartworm caval syndrome
Liver disease

Neoplasia

Increased Hydrostatic Pressure

Vasculitis

Exudate (>5000 Cells, >3.0 Total Solids, >1.025 Specific Gravity)

Nonseptic
Pancreatitis
Feline infectious peritonitis (FIP)
Urine
Bile
Neoplasia

Septic
Bowel perforation
Foreign body

Chyle

Trauma
Neoplasia
Infection
Right-sided heart failure

Blood

Coagulopathy
Trauma
Neoplasia (hemangiosarcoma)
Iatrogenic (postsurgical)

Abdominal Pain, Acute

Gastrointestinal System

Gastrointestinal ulceration
Foreign body
Gastric dilation-volvulus
Gastroenteritis
Obstipation
Colitis
Neoplasia
Adhesions
Intestinal ischemia
Intestinal spasm

Urogenital System

Lower urinary tract infection
Lower urinary tract obstruction
Nonseptic cystitis (idiopathic cystitis—cats)
Prostatitis/prostatic neoplasia
Uroliths/renoliths/ureterolith
Pyelonephritis
Neoplasm
Metritis
Pyometra/uterine rupture
Uterine torsion (rare)
Testicular torsion
Mastitis
Dystocia
Ovarian cyst

Pancreatitis

Spleen

Rupture
Neoplasm

Infection
Torsion

Peritoneum

Peritonitis
• Septic
• Nonseptic (e.g., uroabdomen)
Adhesions
Mesenteric neoplasia, volvulus, inflammation

Hepatobiliary

Hepatitis
Hepatic abscess
Hepatic trauma, rupture
Hepatobiliary neoplasia
Cholelithiasis or cholecystitis
Cholangiohepatitis

Musculoskeletal

Fractures
Intervertebral disk disease
Diskospondylitis
Abscess
Strangulated hernia

Miscellaneous

Adrenalitis (associated with hypoadrenocorticism)
Heavy metal intoxication
Vasculopathy
• Rocky Mountain spotted fever
• Infarct
Autonomic (abdominal) epilepsy
Iatrogenic
• Misoprostol
• Bethanechol
• Postoperative pain

Aggressive Behavior

Cats

Pathophysiologic Causes of Feline Aggression

Rabies
Hyperthyroidism
Seizures (epilepsy, central nervous system inflammation)
Paradoxical effects of therapeutic drugs
  (e.g., benzodiazepines)
Toxins (side effects)

Cognitive dysfunction
Brain neoplasia

Species-Typical Patterns of Feline Aggression
Play
Fear
Petting induced
Interspecies aggression
Redirected
Status/assertiveness
Pain induced/irritable
Maternal
Territorial
Predatory
Idiopathic

Dogs

Pathophysiologic Causes of Canine Aggression
Rabies
Seizure activity
Intracranial neoplasia
Cerebral hypoxia
Neuroendocrine disturbances

Species-Typical Patterns of Canine Aggression
Fear related
Conflict related
Resource guarding
Territorial/protective
Intraspecific (intradog)
Redirected
Predatory
Pain/medical/irritable
Play
Maternal/hormonal
Idiopathic

Alopecia

Inflammatory Alopecia

Traumatic
Allergy (flea, atopy, food)
Parasitic dermatitis (flea, scabies, *Cheyletiella* spp., lice, chiggers, etc.)

Infectious
Pyoderma
Demodicosis
Dermatophytosis

Viral
Leishmaniasis
Malassezia spp.

Immune Mediated

Sebaceous adenitis
Superficial pemphigus
Alopecia areata
Erythema multiforme
Systemic lupus erythematosus (SLE), discoid lupus
　erythematosus (DLE)
Epitheliotrophic lymphoma
Vasculitis

Atrophic

Dermatomyositis
Cutaneous vasculitis
Postvaccinal alopecia
Lymphocytic mural folliculitis
Paraneoplastic exfoliative dermatitis
Pseudopelade

Noninflammatory Alopecia

Hormonal

Hyperadrenocorticism
Iatrogenic Cushing's syndrome
Hypothyroidism
Sex hormone imbalance
Alopecia X
Hyperthyroidism (cat)

Canine and Feline Pinnal Alopecia

Canine Pattern Baldness

Canine Follicular Dysplasia

Tricorrhexis nodosa
Pili torti
Color mutant alopecia
Black hair follicular dysplasia

Feline Congenital/Hereditary

Alopecia universalis (Sphinx)
Congenital hypotrichosis
Hair shaft dysplasia (Abyssinian)
Follicular dysplasia (Cornish rex)
Pili torti

Other

Anagen effluvium
Telogen defluxion

Paraneoplastic alopecia
Cyclic follicular dysplasia (seasonal flank alopecia)
Postclipping alopecia
Cicatricial alopecia
Feline preauricular alopecia
Feline acquired symmetric alopecia
Psychogenic alopecia

Anaphylaxis

Venoms

Insects of Hymenoptera order (bees, hornets, ants)
Spiders (brown recluse, black widow)
Snakes (rattlesnakes, copperheads, water moccasins)
Lizards (Gila monster, Mexican beaded lizard)

Drugs

Antibiotics (penicillins, sulfonamides, lincomycin,
   cephalosporins, aminoglycosides, tetracyclines,
   chloramphenicol, polymyxin B, doxorubicin)
Vaccines
Allergen extracts
Blood products
Parasiticides (dichlorophen, levamisole, piperazine,
   dichlorvos, diethylcarbamazine, thiacetarsamide)
Anesthetics/sedatives (acepromazine, ketamine, barbiturates,
   lidocaine, bupivacaine, narcotics, diazepam)
Nonsteroidal antiinflammatory drugs (NSAIDs)
Hormones (insulin, corticotropin, vasopressin, parathyroid
   hormone, glucocorticoids)
Aminophylline
Asparaginase
Iodinated contrast media
Neostigmine
Amphotericin B
Enzymes (trypsin, chymotrypsin)
Vitamins (vitamin K, thiamine, folic acid)
Dextrans and gelatins
Calcium disodium edetate

Foods

Milk, egg white, shellfish, legumes, citrus fruits, chocolate, grains

Physical Factors

Cold, heat, exercise

Anuria and Oliguria

Prerenal Azotemia

Dehydration/hypovolemia

Acute Renal Failure

One third of cases are anuric, one third are oliguric, and one third are nonoliguric; more likely to be oliguric/anuric with severe renal toxicosis

Toxic: exogenous (drugs, biologic or environmental toxins), endogenous (calcium, pigments)

Infectious: pyelonephritis, leptospirosis, infectious canine hepatitis, borreliosis, sepsis

Ischemia: progression of prerenal azotemia, NSAIDs, vascular disease (avulsion, thrombosis, stenosis), shock, decreased cardiac output, deep anesthesia, extensive surgery, hypothermia, hyperthermia, hyperviscosity (polycythemia vera, multiple myeloma, extensive cutaneous burns, transfusion reaction, disseminated intravascular coagulation (DIC)

Immune mediated: acute glomerulonephritis, systemic lupus erythematosus (SLE), transplant rejection, vasculitis

Neoplasia: lymphoma

Systemic disease with renal manifestations

- Infections (feline infectious peritonitis, borreliosis, babesiosis, leishmaniasis, bacterial endocarditis)
- Pancreatitis
- Sepsis
- Multiple organ failure
- Heart failure
- SLE
- Hepatorenal disease
- Malignant hypertension

Postrenal Azotemia

Obstruction (may appear similar to anuria/oliguria)

Anxiety and Phobias

Fears and Phobias

Fear: apprehension associated with the presence of an object, individual, or object; may be normal or abnormal, depending on context

Phobia: quickly developed, immediate, profound abnormal response to a stimulus leading to catatonia or panic

People
Babies, children, elderly
People in uniform
People who appear different than family members
• Color, height, facial hair
Disabled people
Men or women, depending on circumstance

Animals
Same species
Other species

Noise
Especially gunshots, fireworks, thunder

Places

Anxiety

Separation Anxiety
Initiators
Change in owner's routine
Owner returning to school or work
Move to new home
Visit to new environment
After stay in kennel
New baby, new pet
Medical, cognitive

Common Features of Separation Anxiety
Hyperattached to owner
Signs of anxiety as owner leaves
Problems manifest when owner absent or when pet
unable to gain access to owner
Problem behavior begins shortly after owner leaves
May even occur during short absences
Pet shows exuberant greeting behavior

Generalized Anxiety
Poorly socialized, nervous pet

Ascites

See **Abdominal Effusions and Ascites.**

Ataxia and Incoordination

Forebrain Disease

Typically, mild ataxia and other neurologic signs predominate.
Generalized disease: generalized ataxia

Unilateral disease: contralateral conscious proprioceptive deficits, mild gait disturbance

Postictal paraparesis: transient in nature

Paraparesis may be a side effect of anticonvulsant therapy (especially potassium bromide).

Brain Stem

Hemiparesis or tetraparesis; lesions severe enough to cause paralysis usually result in respiratory arrest.

Vestibular nuclei may be affected, causing vestibular ataxia, head tilt, and nystagmus; distinguish central vestibular disease from peripheral vestibular disease by presence of ipsilateral conscious proprioceptive deficits.

Peripheral Vestibular Disease

Generalized ataxia accompanied by head tilt, rotary or horizontal nystagmus, positional strabismus, and oculovestibular eye movements

Conscious proprioceptive deficits absent

Cerebellum

Lesions cause dysmetria, usually hypermetria.

Unilateral lesions cause ipsilateral signs.

Cervical Spinal Cord

May cause forelimb monoparesis (lesions affecting spinal segments C6-T2), hemiparesis, tetraparesis; may progress to paralysis

Thoracic (T3-L3) Spinal Cord

Mild to marked rear limb ataxia, paraparesis, paraplegia, monoparesis, or monoplegia

Rear limb reflexes exaggerated

Reduced to absent panniculus reflex caudal to lesion

Lumbosacral (L4-S2) Spinal Cord

Mild to marked rear limb ataxia, paraparesis, paraplegia, monoplegia

Reduced to absent rear limb reflexes

May see bladder and anal sphincter hypotonia

Peripheral Nerve

Mild to marked ataxia, paresis, paralysis of one or more limbs

Degenerative, inflammatory, toxic, traumatic neuropathies

Hyporeflexia usually seen

Paresis or paralysis of muscle or muscles innervated by affected nerve

Blindness

Corneal Lesions

Edema (trauma, glaucoma, immune-mediated keratitis such as keratouveitis caused by canine adenovirus-1, endothelial dystrophy, neurotropic keratitis)

Keratoconjunctivitis sicca

Exposure keratitis

Superficial keratitis (pannus)

Corneal melanosis (entropion, ectropion, lagophthalmos, facial nerve paralysis)

Cellular infiltrate (bacterial, viral, fungal)

Dystrophies (lipid, genetic)

Fibrosis (scar)

Aqueous Humor Lesions

Fibrin (anterior uveitis: many causes)

Hypopyon (immune-mediated, neoplastic [lymphosarcoma], infectious [blastomycosis, cryptococcus, histoplasmosis, coccidioidomycosis, toxoplasmosis, FIP, protothecoosis, brucellosis, septicemia])

Hyphema (trauma, blood-clotting deficiencies, ehrlichiosis, rickettsia, systemic hypertension, retinal detachment neoplasia)

Lipid (hyperlipidemia with concurrent anterior uveitis to disrupt the blood-aqueous barrier)

Lens Lesions

Cataracts (genetic, metabolic/diabetic, nutritional, traumatic, toxic, retinal degeneration, hypocalcemia, electric shock, chronic uveitis, lens luxation)

Vitreous Humor Lesions

Hemorrhage (trauma, systemic hypertension, clotting deficiency, neoplasia, retinal detachment)

Hyalitis (numerous infectious diseases such as feline infectious peritonitis, penetrating injury causing cellular infiltrate)

Retinal Lesions

Glaucoma

Sudden acquired retinal degeneration (SARD)

Progressive retinal atrophy

Central progressive retinal atrophy

Toxicity (fluoroquinolone administration in cats)

Systemic hypertension

Retinal detachment

- Exudative/transudative (systemic hypertension, mycoses, rickettsial, toxoplasmosis, viral, bacterial, fungal)
- Neoplasia
- Retinal dysplasia
- Hereditary/congenital (e.g., Collie eye anomaly)

Failure to Transmit Visual Message

Viral infections (canine distemper, feline infectious peritonitis [FIP])
Systemic and ocular mycoses (blastomycosis, cryptococcosis, histoplasmosis, coccidioidomycosis)
Neoplasia
Traumatic avulsion of optic nerve (traumatic proptosis)
Granulomatous meningoencephalitis
Hydrocephalus
Optic nerve hypoplasia
Coloboma
Immune-mediated optic neuritis

Failure to Interpret Visual Message

Canine distemper virus
Feline infectious peritonitis (FIP)
Granulomatous meningoencephalitis
Systemic mycoses
Trauma
Heat stroke
Hypoxia
Hydrocephalus
Hepatoencephalopathy
Neoplasia
Storage diseases
Postictal
Meningitis

Bradycardia, Sinus

Normal variation (fit animal)
Hypothyroidism
Hypothermia
Drugs (tranquilizers, anesthetics, β-blockers, calcium entry blockers, digitalis)
Increased intracranial pressure
Brain stem lesion
Severe metabolic disease (e.g., uremia)
Ocular pressure
Carotid sinus pressure

High vagal tone
Cardiac arrest (before and after)
Sinus node disease

Cachexia and Muscle Wasting

Cachexia

Certain chronic disease processes stimulate the release of cytokines that suppress appetite and stimulate hypercatabolism.

Cardiac disease
End-stage renal disease
Chronic infection
Chronic fever
Chronic inflammation
Neoplasia

Muscle Wasting

Endocrine Disease

Hyperadrenocorticism
Hyperthyroidism
Hyperparathyroidism

Starvation

Underfeeding
Poor-quality feed
Competition for food
Dental disease

Impaired Ability to Use or Retain Nutrients

Maldigestion
Malabsorption
Parasitism
Histoplasmosis
Exocrine pancreatic insufficiency
Diabetes mellitus
Protein-losing nephropathy or gastroenteropathy

Inflammatory Myopathies

Masticatory myositis
Dermatomyositis
Canine idiopathic polymyositis
Feline idiopathic polymyositis

Protozoal Myositis

Toxoplasma gondii
Neospora caninum

Inherited Myopathies

Muscular dystrophy
Hereditary Labrador retriever myopathy

Neurologic Disorders

Spinal and peripheral neuropathies
Disuse atrophy

Compulsive Behavior Disorders

Compulsive Disorders in Dogs

Locomotor

Spinning or tail chasing
Stereotypic pacing/circling/jumping
Fixation; staring/barking/freezing/scratching
Chasing lights, reflections, shadows
Barking; intense/rhythmic/difficult to interrupt
Head bob/tremor/head shaking
Attacking food bowl, attacking inanimate objects

Apparent Hallucinatory

Air biting or fly snapping
Staring, freezing, startled
Star/sky gazing

Self-Injurious or Self-Directed

Tail attacking, mutilation, growl/attack legs or rear
Face rubbing/scratching
Acral lick dermatitis, licking/chewing/barbering
Nail biting
Flank sucking
Checking rear

Oral

Sucking/licking
Pica, rock chewing
Polydipsia/polyphagia
Licking of objects/owners

Compulsive Disorders in Cats

Locomotor

Skin ripple/agitation/running, feline hyperesthesia
Circling
Freezing
Excessive/intense chasing of imaginary objects
Excessive vocalization/howling

Apparent Hallucinatory

Staring at shadows/walls
Startle
Avoiding imaginary objects

Self-Injurious or Self-Directed

Tail attacking, mutilation, growl/attack legs or rear
Face scratching/rubbing
Chewing/licking/barbering/overgrooming
Nail biting
Hyperesthesia

Oral

Wool sucking
Pica
Polydipsia/polyphagia
Licking of objects/owners

Constipation

Dietary Causes

Excessive fiber in dehydrated patient
Ingestion of hair, bones, indigestible materials

Colonic Obstruction

Deviation of rectal canal: perineal hernia
Intraluminal or intramural disorders
- Tumor
- Granuloma
- Cicatrix
- Rectal foreign body
- Congenital stricture

Pseudocoprostasis
Perineal hernia
Extraluminal disorders
- Tumor
- Granuloma
- Abscess
- Healed pelvic fracture
- Prostatomegaly
- Prostatic or paraprostatic cyst
- Sublumbar lymphadenopathy

Behavioral or Environmental Causes

Change in routine
Soiled or absent litter box
Refusal to defecate in house
Inactivity

Drugs

Opiates
Anticholinergics
Sucralfate
Barium

Refusal to Defecate

Pain in rectal or perineal area (perianal fistulas)
Inability to posture to defecate
Orthopedic or neurologic problem

Colonic Weakness

Systemic Disease

Hypercalcemia
Hypokalemia
Hypothyroidism
Chagas disease

Localized Neuromuscular Disease

Spinal cord disease
Pelvic nerve damage
Dysautonomia
Chronic dilatation of colon/irreversible stretching of
colonic musculature

Miscellaneous Causes

Severe dehydration
Idiopathic megacolon (cats)

Coughing

Disorders of Upper Airway

Inflammatory

Pharyngitis
Tonsillitis
Tracheobronchitis
Chronic bronchitis
Allergic bronchitis
Bronchiectasis
Collapsed trachea
Oslerus osleri infection

Neoplastic

Mediastinal
Laryngeal
Tracheal

Allergic
    Bronchial asthma

Other
    Bronchial compression: left atrial enlargement, hilar
        lymphadenopathy
    Foreign body
    Inhalation
    Tracheal stenosis

Disorders of Lower Respiratory Tract

Inflammatory
    Pneumonia
        Bacterial
        Viral: canine distemper virus
        Fungal: blastomycosis, histoplasmosis,
            coccidioidomycosis
        Protozoal: toxoplasmosis, pneumocystis
            pneumonia

    Granuloma, Abscess

    Chronic Pulmonary Fibrosis

Parasitic Disease
    Heartworm disease *(Dirofilaria immitis)*
    Lungworm disease (*Aelurostrongylus abstrusus*—cat;
        Paragonimus kellicotti—dog, cat; *Capillaria aerophilia*—
        dog, cat; *Filaroides hirthi*—dog; *Crenosoma vulpis*—dog;
        Angiostrongylus vasorum—dog)

Neoplasia
    Primary or metastatic
    Lymphoma

Cardiovascular
    Left-sided heart failure: pulmonary edema
    Pulmonary thromboembolism

Noncardiogenic Pulmonary Edema

Allergic
    Eosinophilic pneumonitis
    Eosinophilic pulmonary granulomatosis
    Pulmonary infiltrate with eosinophils (PIE)

Other
    Lung lobe torsion
    Systemic bleeding disorder
    Pleural effusion
    Neoplasia of chest wall

Cyanosis

Central Cyanosis

Cardiac

Intracardiac

Tetralogy of Fallot

Atrial or ventricular septal defect with pulmonic stenosis, tricuspid valve dysplasia, or pulmonary hypertension

Transposition complexes (double outlet right ventricle, other)

Extracardiac

Pulmonary arteriovenous fistulas

Patent ductus arteriosus (reversed)

Pulmonary

Hypoventilation

Pleural effusion

Pneumothorax

Respiratory muscle failure (fatigue, neuromuscular disease)

Anesthetic overdose

Primary neurologic disease

Obstruction

Laryngeal paralysis

Foreign body in airway

Mass lesion of large airway (neoplasia, parasitic, inflammatory)

Low oxygen concentration of inspired air (high altitude, anesthetic complications)

Ventilation-Perfusion Mismatch

Pulmonary thromboembolism

Pulmonary infiltrate (edema, inflammation/infection, neoplasia, acute respiratory distress syndrome, chronic obstructive pulmonary disease, fibrosis, pulmonary contusions/hemorrhage)

Methemoglobinemia

Peripheral Cyanosis

Central cyanosis (heart failure)

Decreased arterial supply

Peripheral vasoconstriction (hypothermia, shock)

Arterial thromboembolism

Low cardiac output

Obstruction of venous drainage

- Tourniquet or foreign object (e.g., rubber band)
- Venous thrombosis
- Right-sided heart failure

Deafness

Congenital Sensorineural Deafness

Inherited

Many breeds of dogs

- Dalmatians
- Merle or dapple coat patterns in Collies, Shetland Sheepdogs, Great Danes, Dachshunds
- Piebald pattern in Dalmatians, Bull Terriers, Great Pyrenees, Sealyham Terriers, Greyhounds, Bulldogs, and Beagles)
- Many other dog breeds affected

White cats with blue irides and white coloration in some breeds of dogs

Congenital Acquired Sensorineural Deafness

In utero exposure to bacteria, ototoxic drugs, low oxygen tensions, or trauma

Acquired Late-Onset Conductive Deafness

Lack of transmission of sound through tympanic membrane and auditory ossicles

Otitis externa/media

Otic neoplasia

Polyps

Trauma-induced fluid accumulation in middle ear

Atresia of tympanum or ossicles

Fused ossicles

Stenosis of ear canal leading to accumulation of fluid in middle ear

Acquired Late-Onset Sensorineural Deafness

Presbycusis (age-related hearing loss)

Ototoxicity

Chronic exposure to loud noise

Hypothyroidism

Trauma

Bony neoplasia

Diarrhea, Acute

Diet

Intolerance/allergy
Rapid dietary change
Bacterial food poisoning
Dietary indiscretion
Poor quality food

Parasites

Helminths
Protozoa (*Giardia, Tritrichomonas,* Coccidia spp.)

Infections

Viral (parvovirus, coronavirus, feline leukemia virus [FeLV],
   feline immunodeficiency virus [FIV], canine distemper
   virus, rotavirus)
Bacterial *(Salmonella* spp., *Clostridium perfringens, Escherichia
   coli, Campylobacter jejuni, Yersinia enterocolitica,* other
   bacteria)
Rickettsial
• Salmon poisoning

Other Causes

Hemorrhagic gastroenteritis
Intussusception
Irritable bowel syndrome
Toxins (chemicals, heavy metals, toxic plants)
Drugs (antibiotics, cancer chemotherapeutic agents,
   anthelmintics, NSAIDs, digitalis, lactulose)
Pancreatitis
Hypoadrenocorticism
Pyometra
Peritonitis

Diarrhea, Chronic

Small Bowel Diarrhea

Food intolerance or allergy
Inflammatory bowel disease
Gastrointestinal lymphoma
Pancreatic exocrine insufficiency
Chronic parasitism (hookworm, *Giardia*)
Histoplasmosis
Intestinal lymphangiectasia
Partial obstruction

Pancreatic carcinoma
Gastrinoma
Liver disease (hepatocellular failure, cholestasis)
Endocrine disease (hypoadrenocorticism, hypothyroidism, hyperthyroidism)
Renal disease (uremia, nephrotic syndrome)
Chronic intussusception
Small intestinal bacterial overgrowth
Pythiosis

Large Bowel Diarrhea

Food intolerance or allergy
Parasitism (whipworm, *Giardia, Tritrichomonas*)
Clostridial colitis
Irritable bowel syndrome
Histoplasmosis
Pythiosis
Inflammatory bowel disease
- Lymphocytic-plasmacytic colitis
- Eosinophilic colitis
- Chronic ulcerative colitis
- Histiocytic ulcerative colitis (boxers)
Neoplasia (lymphoma, adenocarcinoma)
FeLV/FIV (infections secondary to these viruses)

Dyschezia

See **Tenesmus and Dyschezia.**

Dysphagia

Oral Lesions

Fractured bones or teeth
Periodontitis
Trauma (laceration, hematoma)
Feline resorptive lesions (caries)
Osteomyelitis
Retrobulbar abscess/inflammation
Temporal-masseter myositis
Stomatitis, glossitis, pharyngitis, gingivitis, tonsillitis, sialoadenitis
- Immune-mediated disease
- Feline herpesvirus, calicivirus, leukemia virus, immunodeficiency virus
- Lingual foreign bodies or granulomas

- Tooth root abscess
- Uremia
- Caustic chemicals

Cleft palate

Lingual frenulum disorder

Cricopharyngeal achalasia/asynchrony

Obstructive Lesion

Esophageal stricture/foreign object

Esophagitis

Electric cord burns

Neoplasia (malignant or benign)

Inflammatory (abscess, polyp, granuloma)

Lymphadenopathy

Eosinophilic granuloma

Foreign object (oral, pharyngeal, laryngeal)

Sialocele

Nasopharyngeal polyp

Neuromuscular Disease

Myasthenia gravis

Acute polyradiculitis

Masticatory myositis

Tick paralysis

Botulism

Polymyositis

Temporomandibular joint disease

Rabies

Trigeminal nerve paralysis or neuritis

Neuropathies of cranial nerves V, VII, IX, X, or XII

Brain stem disease

Tetanus

Hypothyroidism

Dyspnea

Inspiratory Dyspnea

Nasal Obstruction

Rhinitis

- Viral: feline herpesvirus, feline calicivirus, canine distemper virus
- Bacterial
- Fungal: aspergillosis, cryptococcosis, penicilliosis, rhinosporidiosis

Neoplasia: adenocarcinoma, squamous cell carcinoma,
fibrosarcoma, osteosarcoma, chondrosarcoma, lym-
phoma, transmissible venereal tumor
Stenotic nares
Nasal foreign body
Thick nasal discharge of any etiology

Pharyngeal or Laryngeal Disease
Elongated soft palate, everted laryngeal saccules
Neoplasia/mass, abscess, granuloma, extraluminal mass
Nasopharyngeal polyp
Foreign body
Laryngeal paralysis, acute/obstructive laryngitis, laryngeal
collapse, laryngeal trauma

Extrathoracic Trachea
Collapsing trachea
Tracheal hypoplasia
Tracheal trauma/stricture, foreign body, neoplasia

Expiratory or Mixed Dyspnea

Intrathoracic Trachea and Bronchi
Collapsing trachea or main-stem bronchus
Trauma, stricture, foreign body, neoplasia

Small Airway Disease
Feline asthma
Bronchitis
Smoke inhalation
Bronchopneumonia

Pulmonary Parenchymal Disease
Pneumonia (viral, bacterial, fungal, protozoal, aspiration)
Pulmonary edema
Pulmonary thromboembolism
Bronchial asthma
Chronic obstructive lung disease

Parasites/Severe Infestations/Heartworm, Lungworms
Pulmonary fibrosis
Neoplasia

Pleural Space Disease
Pleural effusion
Pneumothorax
Pleural space masses
Diaphragmatic hernia

Noncardiopulmonary Disease
Severe anemia
Hypovolemia

Acidosis
Hyperthermia
Neurologic disease

Dysuria

See **Stranguria, Dysuria, and Pollakiuria.**

Ecchymoses

See **Petechiae and Ecchymoses.**

Edema

Increased Hydrostatic Pressure

Impaired Venous Return
Congestive heart failure
Constrictive pericarditis
Ascites (cirrhosis)
Budd-Chiari syndrome
Venous obstruction or compression (thrombosis, external
pressure, extremity inactivity)
Iatrogenic overhydration
Heartworm disease

Small-Caliber Arteriolar Dilatation
Heat
Neurohumoral dysregulation

Reduced Plasma Osmotic Pressure

Hypoproteinemia
Cirrhosis (ascites)
Malnutrition
Protein-losing enteropathy
Protein-losing glomerulonephropathy (nephrotic
syndrome)
Lymphangiectasia

Lymphatic Obstruction

Various inflammatory causes
Neoplasia
Postsurgical
After radiation therapy

Sodium Retention

Excessive dietary intake with renal disease
Renal hypoperfusion
Increased renin-angiotension-aldosterone secretion

Inflammation

Acute and chronic
Angiogenesis

Increased Microvascular Permeability

Sepsis
Acute respiratory distress syndrome
Pancreatitis
Infection (fungal, bacterial, viral)

Mixed Mechanisms

Noncardiogenic pulmonary edema (head trauma, seizures, electrocution, upper airway obstruction)
Anaphylaxis
Organ torsion

Epistaxis

Systemic Causes

Thrombocytopenia
- Decreased production of thrombocytes (infectious, myelophthisis secondary to neoplasia, drugs, immune mediated phenomena)
- Increased destruction (immune mediated, microangiopathy)
- Increased consumption (disseminated intravascular coagulation, vasculitis, hemorrhage)

Thrombocytopathia
- Primary (von Willebrand disease)
- Secondary (uremia, ehrlichiosis, multiple myeloma, drugs such as NSAIDs)

Coagulation factor defects (e.g., hemophilia A and B)
Acquired coagulopathies (anticoagulant rodenticides, hepatic failure)
Increased capillary fragility (hypertension, hyperviscosity syndromes, hyperlipidemia, thromboembolic disease)
Polycythemia
Systemic hypertension

Local Causes

Neoplasia (nasal adenocarcinoma, lymphoma, benign polyps)
Bacterial infection (usually secondary; rarely, *Bordetella, Pasteurella,* or *Mycoplasma* can be primary cause of epistaxis)
Fungal rhinitis (*Aspergillus, Cryptococcus* spp.)

Dental disease with oronasal fistulation

Nasal parasites: *Pneumonyssus caninum* (nasal mite), *Eucoleus boehmi* (formerly *Capillaria* spp.), *Cuterebra* spp.

Eosinophilic and lymphoplasmacytic rhinitis (uncommon)

Arteriovenous malformations

Erosions and Ulcers of Skin and Mucous Membranes

Canine Diseases

Infectious
- Bacterial pyoderma
- Surface: Acute moist dermatitis (pyotraumatic dermatitis), intertrigo
- Deep: folliculitis/furunculosis (including pyotraumatic folliculitis), oral bacterial infections

Fungal
- Yeast infections (Malassezia pachydermatis, Candida spp.), systemic/subcutaneous

Parasitic
- Demodecosis

Metabolic
- Calcinosis cutis (hyperadrenocorticism)
- Uremia/renal failure
- Necrolytic migratory erythema/metabolic epidermal necrosis

Neoplastic
- Epitheliotropic lymphoma
- Squamous cell carcinoma

Physical, Chemical
- Drug reactions
- Solar injury
- Thermal injury (freeze, burn)
- Urine scald

Immune-Mediated/Autoimmune
- Discoid lupus erythematosus
- Pemphigus group
- Uveodermatologic syndrome
- Miscellaneous autoimmune subepidermal vesiculobullous diseases: bullous pemphigoid, epidermolysis bullosa acquisita, linear IgA bullous disease, mucocutaneous pemphigoid, bullous systemic lupus-type 1

Miscellaneous
- Arthropod bites
- Dermatomyositis
- Dystrophic epidermolysis bullosa
- Idiopathic ulceration of Collies
- Junctional epidermolysis bullosa
- Toxic epidermal necrolysis/erythema multiforme

Feline Diseases

Infectious
- Viral: calicivirus and herpesvirus
- Bacterial: atypical mycobacteriosis
- Fungal: Subcutaneous and systemic mycoses, cryptococcosis, sporotrichosis

Metabolic
- Uremia/renal disease

Neoplastic
- Fibrosarcoma
- Lymphoma
- Squamous cell carcinoma

Physical/Chemical
- Drug reactions
- Thermal

Immune-Mediated/Autoimmune
- Bullous pemphigoid
- Pemphigus foliaceous
- Toxic epidermal necrolysis/erytherma multiformed

Miscellaneous/Idiopathic
- Arthropod bites
- Dystrophic epidermolysis bullosa
- Eosinophilic plaque
- Idiopathic ulceration of dorsal neck
- Indolent ulcer
- Junctional epidermolysis bullosa

Failure to Grow/Failure to Thrive

Small Stature and Poor Body Condition

Dietary insufficiency
Underfeeding
Poor-quality diet
Gastrointestinal disease
- Parasitism
- Inflammatory bowel disease

- Obstruction (foreign body, intussusception)
- Histoplasmosis

Hepatic dysfunction

- Portovascular anomaly
- Hepatitis
- Glycogen storage disease

Cardiac disorder

- Congenital anomaly
- Endocarditis

Pulmonary disease

Esophageal disease

- Megaesophagus
- Vascular ring anomaly (persistent right aortic arch)

Exocrine pancreatic insufficiency

Renal disease

Renal failure (congenital or acquired)

- Glomerular disease
- Pyelonephritis

Inflammatory disease

Hormonal disease

- Diabetes mellitus
- Hypoadrenocorticism
- Diabetes insipidus
- Juvenile hyperparathyroidism

Small Stature and Good Body Condition

Chondrodystrophy

Hormonal disease

- Congenital hypothyroidism
- Congenital hyposomatotropism (pituitary dwarfism)
- Hyperadrenocorticism

Fever of Unknown Origin

Infection

Bacterial

Abscessation (inapparent subcutaneous, stump pyometra, liver, pancreas)

Pyelonephritis

Diskospondylitis

Prostatitis

Peritonitis

Pyothorax

Closed pyometra

Splenic abscess

Septic arthritis

    Bartonellosis
    Mycoplasma haemofilis (formerly *Hemobartonella felis*)
    Borreliosis
    Bacterial endocarditis
    Plague
    Tuberculosis

Fungal
    Blastomycosis
    Histoplasmosis
    Coccidioidomycosis

Viral
    Feline immunodeficiency virus (FIV)
    Feline leukemia virus (FeLV)
    Feline infectious peritonitis (FIP; *Coronavirus*)

Rickettsial
    Rocky Mountain spotted fever
    Ehrlichiosis
    Salmon poisoning

Protozoal
    Toxoplasmosis
    Babesiosis
    Hepatozoonosis
    Cytauxzoonosis
    Trypanosomiasis (Chagas disease)
    Leishmaniasis

Neoplasia

Lymphoma
Multiple myeloma
Leukemia
Malignant histiocytosis
Necrotic solid tumors

Immune Mediated

Polyarthritis
Vasculitis
Meningitis
SLE
Immune-mediated anemia
Steroid-responsive fever
Steroid-responsive neutropenia

Other

Hyperthyroidism
Tissue damage

Pharmacologic agents
- Tetracycline
- Penicillins
- Sulfas

Metabolic bone disease

Idiopathic

Flatulence

Dietary intolerance (high-fiber, high-protein, or high-fat foods; high-sulfur diets; spoiled food; food change)

Maldigestion
- Exocrine pancreatic insufficiency
- Lactose intolerance

Malabsorption

Motility disorders (disrupt passage of gas)

Aerophagia

Behavior (aerophagia associated with competitive eating habits)

Various gastrointestinal disorders

Gagging

Nutritional

Food texture
Food size

Infectious

Viral encephalitis (rabies, pseudorabies)
Fungal (focal, systemic)
Bacterial encephalitis

Toxic

Chemical (caustic chemicals, smoke)
Botulism

Developmental

Cleft palate
Hydrocephalus
Achalasia

Degenerative

Laryngeal paralysis
Muscular dystrophy
Myasthenia gravis
Neuropathy of cranial nerves V, VII, IX, or XII

Mechanical

Foreign body
Styloid disarticulation

Metabolic

Uremia
Hypocalcemia

Neoplasia

Tonsils, pharynx, epiglottis, glottis, inner ear, nasal, central
nervous system

Trauma

Tracheal rupture
Pharyngeal hematoma
Medulla or pons ischemia or edema

Allergic or Immune Mediated

Rhinitis
Pharyngitis
Laryngitis
Asthma
Granuloma complex
Idiopathic glossopharyngitis

Genital Dermatoses

Lesions of the Prepuce/Sheath

Bacterial folliculitis/furunculosis
Allergic dermatitis affecting the abdomen with
  hyperpigmentation/lichenification/hypertrophy of the
  sheath
Localized demodicosis
Vasculitis
Autoimmune skin diseases
Linear dermatosis of the prepuce (estrogen-secreting tumor)
Linear epidermal nevus
Vascular nevus
Various neoplasms (Stricker sarcoma, hemangiosarcoma,
  mast cell tumor)

Lesions of the Scrotum

Contact dermatitis (most common scrotal skin disease)
Frostbite
Intertrigo
Malassezia dermatitis

Prototothecosis
Babesiosis
Cuterebrosis
Brucellosis
Infection with *Erysipelothrix rhusiopathiae*
Rocky Mountain spotted fever
Autoimmune diseases (bullous diseases, lupus)
Erythema multiforme
Fixed pigmented erythema
Cutaneous histiocytosis
Vascular hamartoma
Neoplasms (squamous cell carcinoma, apocrine adenocarcinoma, myxoma and fibrosarcoma, hemangioma, recurrent cystic hemangioma and hemangiosarcoma, plasmocytoma, lymphoma, histiocytoma, benign fibrous histiocytoma, mast cell tumor, melanoma)

Female

Intertrigo
Allergic dermatitis affecting the abdomen with hyperpigmentation/lichenification/hypertrophy of the vulva
Malassezia dermatitis
Demodicosis
Bacterial furunculosis
Contact dermatitis
Autoimmune diseases (lupus, bullous diseases)
Endocrine disorders (especially hyperestrogenism)
Neoplasms

Halitosis

Oral Disease

Periodontal disease (gingivitis, periodontitis, abscessation)
Calculus
Food traps (periodontal pockets, exposed tooth roots, oral ulcers)
Neoplasia (melanoma, fibrosarcoma, squamous cell carcinoma)
Foreign body
Trauma/fracture
Electric cord injury
Pharyngitis
Stomatitis/glossitis

Metabolic Disease

Renal failure (uremia)
Diabetic ketoacidosis

Gastrointestinal Disease

Megaesophagus
Inflammatory bowel disease
Exocrine pancreatic insufficiency

Respiratory Disease

Rhinitis/sinusitis
Neoplasia
Pneumonia or pulmonary abscess

Dermatologic Disease

Lip fold pyoderma
Eosinophilic granuloma
Pemphigus complex
Bullous pemphigoid
Lupus erythematosus
Drug eruption
Cutaneous lymphoma
Exposure to dimethyl sulfoxide (DMSO)

Dietary

Aromatic foods (onions, garlic)
Fetid food (carrion)
Coprophagy

Grooming Behavior

Anal sacculitis
Vaginitis/balanoposthitis
Lower urinary tract infections
Hair retained in periodontal pockets

Head Tilt

Peripheral Vestibular Disease

Otitis media/interna
Feline idiopathic vestibular disease
Geriatric canine vestibular disease
Feline nasopharygeal polyps
Middle ear tumor
• Ceruminous gland adenocarcinoma
• Squamous cell carcinoma
Trauma
Aminoglycoside ototoxicity

Hypothyroidism (possibly)
Congenital (German Shepherd, Doberman Pinscher, English
   Cocker Spaniel, Siamese and Burmese cats)

Central Vestibular Disease

Trauma/hemorrhage
Infectious inflammatory disease
- Rocky Mountain spotted fever
- Feline infectious peritonitis (FIP)
- Bacterial
- Protozoal
- Mycotic
- Rickettsial
- Others

Granulomatous meningoencephalitis
Neoplasia (meningioma, choroid plexus tumors)
Vascular infarct
Thiamine deficiency
Metronidazole toxicity
Viral (canine distemper virus, FIP)
Toxic (lead, hexachlorophene)
Degenerative diseases (storage diseases, neuronopathies,
   demyelinating diseases)
Hydrocephalus

Hematemesis

Alimentary Tract Lesion

Gastritis

Acute gastritis (common cause)
Hemorrhagic gastroenteritis
Chronic gastritis
Helicobacter-associated disease

Foreign Body

Gastrointestinal Tract Ulceration/Erosion

Iatrogenic

Nonsteroidal antiinflammatory drugs (NSAIDs)
Corticosteroids
NSAIDs used in combination with
   corticosteroids

Infiltrative Disease

Neoplasia
Inflammatory bowel disease
Pythiosis (young dogs, southeastern United States)
Stress ulceration

- Hypovolemic shock
- Septic shock
- After gastric dilatation/volvulus
- Neurogenic shock

Hyperacidity
- Mast cell tumor
- Gastrinoma (rare)

Other causes
- Hepatic disease
- Renal disease
- Hypoadrenocorticism
- Inflammatory disease

Esophageal Disease (Uncommon)

Tumor
Severe esophagitis
Trauma

Bleeding Oral Lesion

Gallbladder Disease (Rare)

Coagulopathy

Thrombocytopenia/platelet dysfunction
Clotting factor deficiency
DIC

Extraalimentary Tract Lesion

Respiratory tract lesion
Lung lobe torsion
Pulmonary tumor
Posterior nares lesion

Hematochezia

Anal Disease

Perianal fistulas
Anal sacculitis or abscess
Stricture
Neoplasia (anal sac adenocarcinoma)
Anal trauma
Perineal hernia
Foreign body

Rectal and Colonic Disease

Hemorrhagic gastroenteritis
Proctitis
Colitis

- Idiopathic
- Dietary allergy
- Inflammatory bowel disease
- Stress
- Infectious (*Campylobacter* spp., *Clostridium perfringens*)
- Histoplasmosis
- Pythiosis

Parvovirus

Parasites
- Whipworms
- Hookworms
- Coccidia

Neoplasia
- Rectal polyp
- Adenocarcinoma
- Lymphoma
- Leiomyoma or leiomyosarcoma

Prolapsed rectum

Mucosal trauma
- Foreign body or foreign material
- Pelvic fractures
- Iatrogenic (thermometers, enemas, fecal loops, rectal palpation)

Iliocecal intussusception

Hematuria

Renal or Lower Urinary Tract Disease

Inflammation/infection
Urolithiasis
Obstruction
Trauma
Neoplasia
Bleeding disorder
Heat stroke
Renal infarct
Granulomatous urethritis
Feline lower urinary tract disease (FLUTD)
Parasitism
Drug induced (cyclophosphamide)
Renal pelvic hematoma
Vascular malformation
Idiopathic renal hematuria
Renal telangiectasia of Welsh Corgis
Renal hematuria of Weimaraners
Pseudohematuria (myoglobin, hemoglobin, drugs, dyes)

Extraurinary Disease

Prostatic disease (infection, tumor, cyst, abscess)
Uterine disease (pyometra, proestrus, tumor, subinvolution
of placental sites)
Vaginal (trauma, neoplasia)
Preputial/penile (trauma, neoplasia)

Hemoptysis

Cardiovascular

Heartworm disease
Cardiogenic pulmonary edema
Arteriovenous fistula
Bacterial endocarditis

Pulmonary

Thromboembolism (secondary to neoplasia, endocrine,
cardiac, metabolic disease)
Bacterial pneumonia
Pulmonary abscess
Nocardiosis
Bordetella bronchiseptica infection
Chronic bronchitis/bronchiectasis
Fungal pneumonia (blastomycosis, coccidiomycosis,
histoplasmosis)
Neoplasia (primary adenocarcinoma, undifferentiated
carcinoma, squamous cell carcinoma, chondrosarcoma,
metastatic or primary tracheal tumors)
Lung lobe torsion
Parasites *(Paragonimus kellicotti, Capillaria aerophila,
Aelurostrongylus abstrusus)*
Pulmonary infiltrate with eosinophils
Systemic bleeding disorder
    Primary (quantitative or qualitative platelet defects)
    Secondary (factor deficiencies, anticoagulant rodenticide
        toxicity, disseminated intravascular coagulopathy)
Trauma (pulmonary contusion, tracheal rupture, foreign body)
Iatrogenic (endotracheal intubation, complication of lung
biopsy/aspirate, transtracheal wash, bronchoscopy)

Hemorrhage, Prolonged

See **Part Two, Section V: Differential Diagnosis for
Thrombocytopenia, Platelet Dysfunction, and Coagulopathies,
Inherited and Acquired.**

Horner Syndrome

2.5% phenylephrine eye drops applied

No Pupillary Dilation (Assume Preganglionic Lesion)

First Order (Central)

Intracranial disease (neoplasia, trauma, infarct)
First cervical to third thoracic (C1-T3) spinal myelopathy
(intervertebral disc disease, neoplasia, fibrocartaginous
embolism, trauma)

Second Order (Preganglionic)

Spinal cord lesion T1-T3 (trauma, neoplasia,
fibrocartilaginous embolism)
Thoracic disease (cranial mediastinal mass, thoracic
spinal nerve root tumor)
Brachial plexus avulsion
Cervical soft-tissue neoplasia, trauma
Skull base tumor
Jugular furrow disease

Pupillary Dilation (Assume Postganglionic Lesion)

Third Order (Postganglionic)

Feline leukemia virus, feline immunodeficiency virus
Otitis media/interna
Otic mass
Retrobulbar injury, neoplasia
Idiopathic

Hyperpigmentation

Increased melanin in the epidermis

Hereditary Hyperpigmentation

Lentigenes—darkly pigmented macules that develop on the
ventral abdomen of healthy adult dogs and on the lips, nose,
gingiva, and eyelids of orange cats. No adverse health effects.
Canine acanthosis nigricans—bilateral hyperpigmentation
and lichenification of axillary skin. Primary, hereditary
form seenin Dachshunds beginning before age 1. When
seen in older Dachshunds or other breeds, it is likely a
postinflammatory form seen with friction, intertrigo,
allergies, or endocrine disease.
Acromelanism—dark areas on the points of Siamese,
Himalayan-Persian, Balinese, and Burmese cats. Result of
a temperature-dependent enzyme controlling melanin
production in hair bulbs.

Acquired Hyperpigmentation

Postinflammatory—Mediators of inflammation (e.g., leukotrienes, thromboxanes) stimulate melanocytes to increase melanin production, which down regulates inflammation by scavenging free radicles. Examples of inflammatory conditions that lead to increased melanin production include allergies, Malassezia dermatitis, bacterial pyoderma, dermatophytosis, demodecosis, scabies, and actinic and intertrigo dermatitis. Inflammation affecting hair follicles may lead to melanotrichia (e.g., sebaceous adenitis, panniculitis, vaccine reactions).

Endocrine—hyperadrenocorticism, hypoadrenocorticism, hypothyroidism, hyperestrogenism, and other sex hormone imbalances may result in diffuse hyperpigmentation.

Papillomavirus associated—Pugs may be at risk for development of papillomavirus-associated, slightly raised, scaly, hyperpigmented macules and plaques in their groin region, abdomen, ventral thorax, and neck. Similar lesions are described in miniature Schnauzers, American Staffordshire terriers, and Pomeranians. May transform to squamous cell carcinoma.

Pigmented tumors—apocrine cysts are bluish, cutaneous hemangiomas and hemangiosarcomas appear red, dark purple, or bluish-black. Melanomas, melanocytomas, and basal cell tumors are frequently black. Squamous cell carcinomas, trichoblastomas, and fibromas also may be dark brown to black.

Hyperthermia

Fever

Exogenous pyrogens (infectious agents and their products, inflammation or necrosis of tissue, immune complexes, pharmacologic agents, bile acids)
Endogenous pyrogens (fever-producing cytokines)

Heat Stroke

High ambient temperatures
Exercise
Poor ventilation
Brachycephalic conformation
Obesity

Exercise Hyperthermia

Sustained exercise
Seizure disorders (especially prolonged or cluster seizures)
Hypocalcemic tetany (eclampsia)

Pathologic Etiologies

Lesions in or around anterior hypothalamus
Hypermetabolic disorders

Hyperthyroidism
Pheochromocytoma
Malignant hyperthermia
Halothane
Succinylcholine

Hypopigmentation

Due to melanocyte destruction, dysfunction, or abnormal distribution of melanosomes.

Hereditary Hypopigmentation

Albinism—hereditary absence of pigment

Piebaldism—presence of white spots where melanocytes are absent

Waardenburg-Klein syndrome—affected animals have absence of melanocytes in areas of skin and hair, blue or heterochromatic eyes, and are also deaf. Reported in cats, bull terriers, Sealyham terriers, collies, Dalmatians

Canine cyclic hematopoiesis—lethal autosomal recessive disease of collies. Gray coat, light-colored nose, cyclic episodes of neutropenia every 12-14 days resulting in sepsis and amyloidosis

Chédiak-Higashi syndrome—rare autosomal recessive disease of blue smoke Persian cats. Partial oculocutaneous albinism with abnormal function of granulocytes and platelets resulting in hemorrhage, recurrent infections, and death at a young age.

Graying—age-associated, reduction of melanocyte replication.

Vitiligo—macular leukoderma and leukotrichia of nose, ears, buccal mucosa, and facial skin. Antimelanocyte antibodies found in serum of some affected dogs. Seen most commonly in Siamese cat, Belgian Tervuren, German Shepherd, collie, Rottweiler, Doberman Pinscher, Giant Schnauzer.

Nasal hypopigmentation—season-associated lightening of nasal planum during winter months most common in Siberian Husky, Golden Retriever, Labrador Retriever, and Bernese Mountain Dog. Seen also in many other breeds.

Acquired Hypopigmentation

Postinflammatory—Discoid lupus erythematosus is the most common cause of postinflammatory nasal depigmentation. Also pemphigus complex, SLE, uveodermatologic syndrome, bullous pemphigoid, mucocutaneous pyoderma, drug eruption, and contact dermatitis. Infectious causes include leishmaniasis, blastomycosis, sporotrichosis, and bacterial folliculitis.

Drug related—ketoconazole, procainamide, and vitamin E may cause diffuse coat lightening.

Nutritional/metabolic—deficiencies of zinc, pyridoxine, pantothenic acid, and lysine are associated with graying of hair. Dark hairs may become reddish in color with copper deficiency, hypothyroidism, hyperadrenocorticism, hyperestrogenism, hyperprogesteronism, chlorine exposure, and chronic exposure to ultraviolet light.

Neoplasia associated—nasal depigmentation, leukoderma, and leukotrichia sometimes seen with epitheliotropic T cell lymphoma, basal cell tumors, mammary adenocarcinoma, and gastric carcinomas.

Idiopathic—leukotrichia and patchy hypopigmentation reported as idiopathic in Labrador Retrievers, and black Newfoundlands. Siamese cats may be affected with periocular leukotrichia, which may be associated with upper respiratory tract infections, pregnancy, dietary deficiencies, or systemic illness.

Hypothermia

Predisposing Factors

Anesthesia
Low ambient temperature
Neonate
Small size
Elderly
Sick
Debilitated
Near drowning
Enema

Icterus (Jaundice)

Hemolysis

Autoimmune hemolytic anemia
Hemolytic anemia secondary to drugs, neoplasia
Infectious (*Ehrlichia canis, Babesia canis, Babesia felis, Mycoplasma hemocanis, Mycoplasma hemofelis, Cytauxzoon felis,* heartworm disease, feline leukemia virus [FELV])
Toxic (onions, lead, copper, methylene blue, benzocaine, proplylene glycol, acetaminophen [cats], phenazopyridine)
Fragmentation (disseminated intravascular coagulation, hemangiosarcoma, vena cava syndrome)
Erythrocyte membrane or enzyme defects (pyruvate kinase deficiency [Beagle, Basenji], phosphofructokinase deficiency [English Springer Spaniel], stomatocytosis of chondrodysplastic Malamutes)

Congenital porphyria
Snake, brown recluse spider, and bee venoms

Hepatobiliary Disease

Cholangiohepatitis
Chronic inflammatory hepatic disease
Cirrhosis
Diffuse neoplasia
Copper toxicity
Toxic hepatopathy (anticonvulsants, mebendazole,
   oxibendazole, diethylcarbamazine, inhalation anesthetics,
   thiacetarsamide, acetaminophen, trimethoprim-sulfa)
Hepatic lipidosis
Feline infectious peritonitis (FIP)
Parasitic
Idiosyncratic drug reaction

Posthepatic Biliary Obstruction

Pancreatitis
Enteritis/cholecystitis
Trauma
Neoplasia
Calculus
Stricture
Mucocele
Ruptured bile duct or gallbladder

Inappropriate Elimination

Dogs

Medical Causes
Fecal House Soiling
Increased volume of feces (maldigestion,
   malabsorption, high-fiber diets)
Increased frequency of voiding (colitis, diarrhea)
Compromised neurologic function (peripheral nerve
   impairment, spinal cord disease, brain tumor,
   encephalitis, infection, degenerative brain disorders)
Joint pain
Sensory decline
Cognitive dysfunction

Urinary House Soiling
Diseases causing polyuria (e.g., renal disease,
   hyperadrenocorticism, diabetes, pyometra)
Increased urinary frequency (urinary tract infection/
   inflammation, urolithiasis, bladder tumors,
   prostatitis, abdominal masses)

Impaired bladder control (peripheral nerve disease,
   spinal cord disease, brain tumor, encephalitis,
   infection, degenerative brain disorders)
Urethral incompetence
Anatomic problems
Urethral sphincter mechanism incompetence
   (estrogen-responsive incontinence)
Cognitive dysfunction

Behavioral Causes
Inadequate training
Submissive urination
Excitement urination
Marking
Separation anxiety
Management-related problems
Location or surface preference

Cats

Medical Causes
Fecal House Soiling
Increased volume of feces (maldigestion,
   malabsorption, high-fiber diets)
Increased frequency of voiding (colitis, diarrhea,
   inflammatory bowel disease)
Compromised neurologic function (peripheral nerve
   impairment, spinal cord disease, brain tumor,
   encephalitis, infection, degenerative brain disorders)
Joint pain
Anal sacculitis
Obstipation/constipation
Hyperthyroidism
Neoplasia
Cognitive dysfunction

Urinary House Soiling
Diseases causing polyuria (e.g., renal disease,
   hyperadrenocorticism, diabetes, pyometra)
Increased urinary frequency (feline lower urinary tract
   disease [FLUTD], urolithiasis, idiopathic cystitis)
Impaired bladder control (peripheral nerve disease,
   spinal cord disease, brain tumor, encephalitis,
   infection, degenerative brain disorders)
Joint pain, disk disease
Hyperthyroidism
Neoplasia
Anatomic problems
Cognitive dysfunction

Behavioral Causes

Litterbox Aversion
Aversive disorder (deodorant, ammonia)
Inadequate cleaning
Discomfort during elimination (FLUTD, constipation, diarrhea, arthritis)
Unacceptable litter (texture, depth, odor, plastic liner)
Unacceptable box (too small, sides too high, covered)
Disciplined, medicated, or frightened in box

Location Aversion
Too much traffic
Traumatic/fearful experience in area

Other
Location preference
Surface preference
Anxiety (owner absence, high cat density, moving, new furniture, inappropriate punishment, teasing, household changes, remodeling in home)
Need for privacy (other pets, anything that makes box less accessible to cat)

Urine Marking
Hormones
Temperament
Feline population density
Indirect signaling from other cats (scent on visitor's clothing)
Changes in environment (new roommate, remodeling home, new furniture, and other novel items in home)
Owner absence from home
Lack of owner attention
Inappropriate punishment

Incontinence, Fecal

Nonneurologic Disease

Colorectal Disease
Inflammatory bowel disease
Neoplasia
Constipation

Anorectal Disease
Perianal fistula
Neoplasia
Surgery (anal sacculectomy, perianal herniorrhaphy, rectal resection and anastomosis)

Miscellaneous
Decreased mentation
Old age
Severe diarrhea
Irritable bowel disease

Neurologic Disease

Sacral Spinal Cord Disease
Diskospondylitis
Neoplasia
Degenerative myelopathy
Congenital vertebral malformation
Sacrococcygeal hypoplasia of Manx cats
Sacral fracture
Sacrococcygeal subluxation
Lumbosacral instability
Meningomyelocele
Viral meningomyelitis

Peripheral Neuropathy
Trauma
Penetrating wounds
Repair of perineal hernia
Perineal urethrostomy
Hypothyroidism
Diabetes mellitus
Dysautonomia

Incontinence, Urinary

Bladder Distended

Neurogenic
Lower motor neuron disease (sacral [S1-S3] segments or
    peripheral nerves)
Bladder easily expressed, dribbles urine
Detrusor areflexia with sphincter areflexia
Upper motor neuron disease
Bladder difficult to express; may be associated with
    paresis, paralysis
Detrusor areflexia with sphincter hypertonia
Dysautonomia

Obstructive
Reflex dyssynergia (functional obstruction)
Mechanical obstruction (uroliths, tumors, strictures,
    granulomatous urethritis, urethral inflammation,
    prostatic disease, mucoid or crystalline plug [feline])

Bladder Not Distended

Dysuria/Pollakiuria Absent

Urethral sphincter mechanism incompetence
(middle-aged to older spayed or neutered dogs)
Congenital (ectopic ureters, patent urachus)

Dysuria/Pollakiuria Present

Detrusor hyperreflexia/instability (uroliths, urinary tract
infection, urethral mass)

Infertility, Female

Normal Cycles

Improper breeding management
Infertile male
Elevated diestrual progesterone
• Early embryonic death
• Lesions in tubular system (vagina, uterus, uterine
tubes)
• Placental lesions (brucellosis, herpes infection)
Normal diestrual progesterone
• Cystic follicles (ovulation failure)

Abnormal Cycles

Abnormal Estrus

Will Not Copulate

Not in estrus
Inexperience
Partner preference
Vaginal anomaly
Hypothyroidism?

Prolonged Estrus

Cystic follicles
Ovarian neoplasia
Exogenous estrogens
Prolonged proestrus

Short Estrus

Observation error
Geriatric
Split estrus

Abnormal Interestrual Interval

Prolonged Interval

Photoperiod (queen)
Pseudopregnant/pregnant (queen)

Normal breed variation
Glucocorticoids (bitch)
Geriatric
Luteal cysts

Short Interval
Normal (especially queen)
Ovulation failure (especially queen)
Corpus luteum failure
"Split heat" (bitch)
Exogenous drugs

Not Cycling

Prepubertal
Ovariohysterectomy
Estrus suppressants
Silent heat
Unobserved heat
Photoperiod (queen)
Intersex (bitch)
Ovarian dysgenesis
Hypothyroidism (possibly)
Glucocorticoid excess
Hypothalamic-pituitary disorder
Geriatric
Ovarian neoplasia
Premature ovarian failure

Infertility, Male

Inflammatory Ejaculate

Prostatitis
Orchitis
Epididymitis

Azoospermia

Sperm-rich fraction not collected
Sperm not ejaculated
• Incomplete ejaculation
• Obstruction
• Prostate swelling
Sperm not produced
• Endocrine
• Testicular
• Metabolic

Abnormal Motility/Morphology

Iatrogenic
Prepubertal
Poor ejaculation
Long abstinence

Abnormal Libido

Female not in estrus
Behavioral
Pain
Geriatric

Normal Libido

Improper stud management
Infertile female

Normal Libido/Abnormal Mating Ability

Orthopedic
Neurologic
Prostatic disease
Penile problem
Prepuce problem

Joint Swelling

Trauma
Degenerative joint disease
Neoplasia
Inflammatory joint disease—infectious
- Septic (bacterial)
- Fungal arthritis
  - Blastomycosis
  - Coccidioidomycosis
  - Cryptococcosis
- Lyme borreliosis
- Rickettsial arthritis
- Mycoplasma
- Bacterial L-form–associated arthritis (cats)
- Viral arthritis (calicivirus infection—kittens)
Inflammatory joint disease—noninfectious
- Nonerosive
  - Immune-mediated polyarthritis (idiopathic)
  - SLE
  - Breed-specific polyarthritis syndromes
  - Akita, Boxer, Weimaraners, Bernese Mountain Dog, German Shorthaired Pointer, Beagle, Shar-Pei

- Lymphocytic/plasmacytic synovitis
- Drug reaction (e.g., trimethoprim-sulfadiazine in Doberman Pinschers)
- Chronic infection causing secondary immune-mediated polyarthritis (bacterial, ehrlichiosis,
- Anaplasmosis, Rocky Mountain spotted fever, Lyme borreliosis, heartworm disease)
- Erosive
  - Rheumatoid arthritis
  - Erosive polyarthritis of greyhounds
  - Feline chronic progressive polyarthritis

Lameness

Orthopedic

Trauma
Fracture
Luxation, subluxation
Toenail trauma
Bone contusion

Infectious
Osteomyelitis (bacterial, fungal)

Developmental
Patellar luxation
Osteochondrosis
Panosteitis
Hypertrophic osteodystrophy
Avascular necrosis of femoral head
Nonunited anconeal process
Bone cysts

Nutritional
Vitamin D deficiency (rickets)

Neoplasia
Osteosarcoma
Multiple myeloma
Metastatic to bone

Joint Disease

See **Joint Swelling.**

Muscles

Trauma
Contusion
Strain

Laceration
Rupture

Inflammatory
Canine idiopathic polymyositis
Feline idiopathic polymyositis
Dermatomyositis

Infectious
Protozoal myositis

Tendons

Trauma
Laceration
Severance
Avulsion

Ligaments

Trauma
Rupture
Tear
Hyperextension

Lymphadenopathy (Lymph Node Enlargement)

Infiltrative Lymphadenopathies

Neoplastic
Primary hemolymphatic (lymphoma, multiple myeloma, systemic mast cell disease, leukemias, malignant histiocytosis, lymphomatoid granulomatosis)
Metastatic neoplasia (carcinomas, sarcomas, malignant melanoma, mast cell tumors)

Nonneoplastic
Eosinophilic granuloma complex
Nonneoplastic mast cell infiltration

Proliferative and Inflammatory Lymphadenopathies

Infectious
Bacterial
- Localized bacterial infection
- Septicemia
- Systemic infection (e.g., *Borrelia burgdorferi, Brucella canis, Yersinia pestis, Corynebacterium, Mycobacterium, Nocardia, Streptococcus, Actinomyces, Bartonella* spp.)
- Contagious streptococcal lymphadenopathy

Parasitic (toxoplasmosis, demodicosis, babesiosis, cytauxzoonosis, hepatozoonosis, leishmaniasis, trypanosomiasis, *Neospora caninum*)

Rickettsial (ehrlichiosis, Rocky Mountain spotted fever, anaplasmosis, salmon poisoning)

Viral (feline immunodeficiency virus, feline leukemia virus, feline infectious peritonitis, canine viral enteritis, infectious canine hepatitis)

Fungal (blastomyosis, cryptococcosis, histoplasmosis, aspergillosis, coccidioidomycosis, phaeohyphomycosis, phycomycosis, sporotrichosis, others)

Algal (prototechosis) *Pneumocystis carinii*

Noninfectious

Immune-mediated disorders
- SLE
- Rheumatoid arthritis
- Immune-mediated polyarthritis
- Juvenile cellulitis

Drug reactions

Localized inflammation

Postvaccinal

Dermatopathic lymphadenopathy

Idiopathic
- Distinctive peripheral lymph node hyperplasia
- Plexiform vascularization of lymph nodes

Melena

Ingested Blood

Oral lesions
Nasopharyngeal lesions
Pulmonary lesions
Diet

Parasitism

Hookworms

Neoplasia

Adenocarcinoma
Lymphoma
Leiomyoma or leiomyosarcoma
Mast cell tumor
Gastrinoma

Upper Gastrointestinal Inflammation

Acute gastritis
Gastroduodenal ulceration/erosion

Hemorrhagic gastroenteritis
Inflammatory bowel disease
Foreign body
Esophagitis

Infection

Campylobacter
Clostridium perfringens
Salmonella
Parvovirus
Neorickettsia helminthoeca (salmon poisoning)
Histoplasma
Pythium

Drugs

Nonsteroidal antiinflammatory drugs (NSAIDs)
Glucocorticoids

Miscellaneous

Pancreatitis
Liver failure
Renal failure
Hypoadrenocorticism
Gastrointestinal ischemia (shock, volvulus, intussusception)
Arteriovenous fistula
Polyps
Coagulopathies (thrombocytopenia, factor deficiencies,
  rodenticide toxicity, DIC)

Muscle Wasting

See **Cachexia and Muscle Wasting.**

Nasal Discharge

See **Sneezing and Nasal Discharge.**

Nystagmus

Peripheral Vestibular Disease

Horizontal nystagmus; fast phase toward normal side; no change
with varying head position
  Otitis media/interna
  Feline idiopathic vestibular disease
  Canine geriatric vestibular disease
  Neoplasia
  Granuloma
  Trauma (iatrogenic secondary to ear cleaning)

Ototoxic drugs
Neuropathy (hypothyroid, cranial nerve VIII disease)
Congenital (German Shepherd, English Cocker Spaniel,
  Doberman Pinscher, smooth-haired Fox Terrier, Siamese,
  Burmese, Tonkinese)

Central Vestibular Disease

Horizontal, vertical, or rotary nystagmus; direction may change
with varying head position
Trauma/hemorrhage
Infectious inflammatory disease
Viral (canine distemper virus, feline infectious peritonitis)
Rickettsial (RMSF, ehrlichiosis)
Fungal (cryptococcosis)
Toxoplasmosis
Neosporosis
Granulomatous meningoencephalitis
Neoplasia
Vascular infarct
Thiamine deficiency
Metronidazole toxicity
Toxic (lead, hexachlorophene)
Degenerative diseases (storage diseases, neuronopathies,
  demyelinating diseases)
Hydrocephalus
Anomaly (caudal occipital malformation syndrome in
  Cavalier King Charles Spaniels)
Head trauma

Obesity

Causes

Excessive feeding
Malnutrition
High-carbohydrate diet (especially cats)
Lack of exercise
Inactivity (indoor life style, middle age)
Neutering?
Genetic predisposition
Hypothyroidism
Hyperadrenocorticism
Hyperinsulinism
Acromegaly
Hypopituitarism
Hypothalamic dysfunction
Drugs (glucocorticoids, progestagens, phenobarbital, primidone)

Health Risks

Degenerative joint disease
Cruciate ligament disease
Hip dysplasia
Traumatic joint disease
Intervertebral disk disease
Dyspnea: (Pickwickian syndrome)
Heat intolerance
Exercise intolerance
Diabetes mellitus (insulin resistance)
Hepatic lipidosis (cats)
Pancreatitis
Dystocia
Urinary tract disease
Skin fold dermatoses
Increased anesthetic risk

Oliguria

See **Anuria and Oliguria.**

Pallor

Anemia

Regenerative Anemia

Immune-mediated hemolytic anemia (extravascular, intravascular)
Erythrocytic parasites (*Bartonella, Babesia, Cytauxzoon* spp.)
Fragmentation (disseminated intravascular coagulation, heartworm disease, hemangiosarcoma, vasculitis, hemolytic uremic syndrome, diabetes mellitus)
Pyruvate kinase deficiency
Phosphofructokinase deficiency
Feline porphyria
Copper toxicity
Neonatal isoerythrolysis
Oxidative injury (onions, acetaminophen, zinc, benzocaine, mothballs, phenazopyridine)
Blood loss (external blood loss, blood loss to a body cavity, coagulopathies, endoparasites, gastrointestinal blood loss)

Nonregenerative Anemia

Anemia of chronic disease
Anemia from renal failure

Feline leukemia virus (FeLV)
Endocrine (mild anemia associated with
 hypoadrenocorticism, hypothyroidism)
Myeloaplasia/aplastic anemia (FeLV infection,
 ehrlichiosis, trimethoprim-sulfa, estrogen toxicity,
 phenylbutazone, chemotherapy, chloramphenicol)
Myelodysplasia
Myeloproliferative and lymphoproliferative disorders
Myelofibrosis

Shock

Cardiogenic

Decreased ventricular function
- Dilated cardiomyopathy
- Myocarditis
- Myocardial infarction

Compromised ventricular filling
- Hypertrophic cardiomyopathy
- Cardiac tamponade

Severe endocardiosis
Outflow obstruction
- Intracardiac tumors
- Aortic stenosis
- Hypertrophic obstructive cardiomyopathy
- Heartworm disease
- Thrombosis
- Severe arrhythmia

Noncardiogenic

Trauma
Hypovolemia
- Severe blood loss
- Dehydration
- Hypoadrenocorticism

Disruptions in blood flow
- Sepsis and endotoxemia
- Hypotension

Papules and Pustules

- Bacterial pyoderma (papules and pustules)
- Demodicosis (papules and pustules)
- Dermatophytosis (rare papules, uncommon pustules)
- Sarcoptes mange (papules, no pustules)
- Cheyletiellosis (rare papules, no pustules)
- Otacariosis (rare papules, no pustules)

- Trombiculosis (papules, rare pustules)
- Hypersensitivity (papules, rare pustules)
- Pemphigus (papules and pustules)
- Early-stage neoplasia (papules, no pustules)

Paresis and Paralysis

Upper Motor Neuron

Tetraparesis or hemiparesis
- Severe forebrain lesion
- Brain stem lesion
- First to fifth cervical (C1-C5) spinal lesion
Paraparesis or rear limb monoparesis
- Third thoracic to third lumbar (T3-L3) spinal lesion

Lower Motor Neuron

Tetraparesis
Generalized lower motor neuron disease
- Flaccid paresis/paralysis
  - Acute polyradiculoneuritis/"coonhound paralysis"
  - Tick paralysis
  - Botulism
  - Myasthenia gravis
- Toxicants
  - Coral snake
  - Black widow spider
  - Herbicides (2,4 D)
  - Macadamia nuts
Paraparesis
- Fourth lumbar to second sacral (L4-S2) spinal lesion
Hemiparesis with lower motor neuron forelimb
- Sixth cervical to second thoracic (C6-T2) spinal lesion
Aortic thromboembolism
Degenerative myelopathy
Monoparesis
Peripheral nerve lesion

Petechiae and Ecchymoses

Thrombocytopenia

Increased Platelet Destruction
Immune-mediated thrombocytopenia
Systemic lupus erythematosus (SLE)
Heartworm disease

Decreased Platelet Production
Bone Marrow Suppression
Infectious disease (ehrlichiosis, babesiosis, Rocky
Mountain spotted fever, leishmaniasis, feline
leukemia virus, feline immunodeficiency virus)
Neoplasia
Drug reactions
Myeloproliferative disease
Virus-associated myelodysplasia
Estrogen toxicity

Consumption of Platelets
Disseminated intravascular coagulation (DIC)
Vasculitis

Sequestration of Platelets (Unlikely to Cause Clinical Signs)
Splenomegaly
Hepatomegaly
Endotoxemia

Thrombopathia

Inherited
Cocker Spaniel, Otterhound, Great Pyrenees, Bassett
Hound, American Cocker Spaniel, cats

Acquired
Drugs (aspirin, cephalothin, carprofen, hydroxyethyl
starch)
Uremia
Liver disease
Dysproteinemias

Von Willebrand Disease
Lack of von Willebrand factor leads to impaired platelet
adhesion.

Vascular Purpura

Vasculitis secondary to infectious, inflammatory, immune-
mediated, neoplasia, drug reaction, hyperadrenocorticism

Pollakiuria

See **Stranguria, Dysuria, and Pollakiuria.**

Polyuria and Polydipsia

Renal insufficiency or failure
Diabetes mellitus

Hyperadrenocorticism (Cushing syndrome)
Lower urinary tract disease
- Infection
- Urolithiasis
- Neoplasia
- Anatomic problem
- Neurologic problem

Pyometra
Hypercalcemia
Hypoadrenocorticism (Addison disease)
Pyelonephritis
Hypokalemia
Iatrogenic (corticosteroids, diuretics, anticonvulsants)
Hyperthyroidism
Hepatic insufficiency
Postobstructive
Diabetes insipidus
- Central
- Renal

Psychogenic drinking
Renal glycosuria

Pruritus

Allergy

Flea allergy
Atopic dermatitis
Food allergy/intolerance
Contact dermatitis
Mosquito-bite hypersensitivity
Eosinophilic plaque (cats)

Parasites

Flea infestation
Scabies
Pediculosis (lice)
Cheyletiellosis
Chiggers
Cutaneous larval migrans
Demodicosis (often not pruritic)
Otodectic acariasis

Infectious Agents

Pyoderma
Malassezia dermatitis
Dermatophytosis

Behavioral

Acral lick dermatosis
Psychogenic alopecia

Immune-Mediated

Pemphigus foliaceus

Drug Eruption

Miscellaneous

Cornification defects
Superficial necrolytic dermatitis
Tail dock neuroma
Rhabditic dermatitis

Ptyalism (Excessive Salivation)

Oral Cavity Disease

Oral trauma (tooth fractures, mandibular fractures, maxillary
fractures, TMJ luxation)
Severe periodontal disease
Oral masses (neoplasia, granuloma, eosinophilic granuloma)
Stomatitis (toxins, infections, immune-mediated disease,
immunologic or nutritional deficiency)
Glossitis (chemical or environmental irritants, viral
infections, uremia, immune-mediated disease, tumors)
Faucitis (cats)
Mucocutaneous junction lesions
Foreign body
Developmental (severe brachygnathism, lip fold pyoderma)

Oral Cavity Normal

Drugs and toxins (bitter taste; insecticides such as
organophosphates, pyrethrins, and D-limonene; caustic
chemicals; poison toads and salamanders)
Nausea
Hepatic encephalopathy/portosystemic shunt
Seizures
Space-occupying lesions in pharynx
Cranial nerve (CN) deficits (CN V: inability to close mouth;
CN VII: inability to move lip; CNs X, XI, and XII: loss of
gag lesion and inability to swallow)
Rabies virus
Dysphagia
Behavior (associated with food [Pavlovian], contentment/
mood in cats when purring, pain)
Salivary gland hypersecretion

Regurgitation

Esophageal Disease

Megaesophagus (primary or secondary)
Esophagitis
Mechanical obstruction (foreign body, vascular ring
anomaly, stricture)

Alimentary Disorders

Pyloric outflow obstruction
Gastric dilatation/volvulus
Hiatal hernia

Neuropathies

Peripheral neuropathy (polyradiculitis, polyneuritis, lead
poisoning, giant cell axonal neuropathy)
Central nervous system (brain stem lesion, neoplastic,
traumatic, distemper)
Dysautonomia

Neuromuscular Junction Abnormalities

Myasthenia gravis (focal or generalized)
Tetanus
Botulism
Acetylcholinesterase toxicity

Immune-Mediated Disorders

Systemic lupus erythematosus (SLE)
Polymyositis
Dermatomyositis

Endocrine Disease

Hypothyroidism
Hypoadrenocorticism

Infectious

Spirocercosis
Pythium insidiosum

Reverse Sneezing

- Loud inspiratory noise, occurs in paroxysms; initiated by
nasopharyngeal irritation
- Purpose is to move secretions and foreign material into the
oropharynx to be swallowed

- Causes include excitement, foreign bodies, nasal mites *(Pneumonyussus caninum)*, viral infections, and epiglottic entrapment of the soft palate
- Often idiopathic, nonprogressive, and common in small dogs and cats

Scaling and Crusting

Bacterial

Superficial folliculitis
Deep pyoderma
Mucocutaneous pyoderma
Pyotraumatic dermatitis

Fungal

Dermatophytosis
Malassezia dermatitis
Deep fungal infection (e.g., blastomycosis, cryptococcosis)

Parasitic

Fleas
Scabies
Demodecosis
Cheyletiellosis
Notoedric mange
Pediculosis

Protozoal

Leishmaniasis

Viral

Feline leukemia virus

Allergic

Atopic dermatitis
Food hypersensitivity
Flea bite hypersensitivity
Military dermatitis

Endocrine and Metabolic

Hyperadrenocorticism
Hypothyroidism
Necrolytic migratory erythema

Immune-Mediated

Pemphigus foliaceus
Discoid lupus erythematosus
Erythema multiforme

Congenital and Hereditary

Primary seborrhea
Ichthyosis
Schnauzer comedo syndrome
Familial canine dermatomyositis

Keratinization Defects

Secondary seborrhea
Vitamin-A responsive dermatosis
Ear margin dermatosis

Environmental

Solar dermatitis

Nutritional

Zinc-responsive dermatosis
Fatty acid deficiency

Other

Cutaneous lymphoma
Sebaceous adenitis
Otitis externa

Seizure

Extracranial Causes

Toxins (e.g., strychnine, chlorinated hydrocarbons,
   organophosphates, carbamates, lead, ethylene glycol,
   metaldehyde)
Metabolic disease (e.g., hepatic encephalopathy,
   hypoglycemia, hypocalcemia)
Hepatic disease
Electrolyte disturbances (e.g., hypernatremia)
Severe uremia
Hyperlipoproteinemia
Hyperviscosity (multiple myeloma, polycythemia)
Hyperosmolality (diabetes mellitus)
Heat stroke

Intracranial Causes

See **Part Two, Section XI: Differential Diagnosis for
Inflammatory Disease of the Nervous System.**

Infectious disease
Neoplasia (primary brain tumor, lymphoma, metastatic
   tumors)
Granulomatous meningoencephalitis

Hemorrhage/infarct (renal failure, hypothyroidism,
  hyperthyroidism, hypertension, septic emboli, neoplasia,
  coagulopathies, heartworm disease, vasculitis)
Congenital malformations (lissencephaly,
  hydrocephalus)
Necrotizing encephalitis
Degenerative diseases (metabolic storage diseases,
  leukodystrophies, hypomyelination disorders, spongy
  disorders)

Idiopathic Epilepsy

Sneezing and Nasal Discharge

Nasal and Upper Respiratory Disease

Infectious

Viral: herpesvirus, calicivirus, canine distemper virus
Bacterial: *Mycoplasma* spp., *Bordatella bronchiseptica*
Fungal: *Aspergillus, Cryptococcus, Rhinosporidium,*
  Penicillium spp.
Parasitic: *Pneumonyssus caninum* (nasal mite), *Eucoleus*
  boehmi (formerly *Capillaria* spp.), *Cuterebra* spp.

Inflammatory

Allergic rhinitis
Lymphocytic-plasmacytic rhinitis
Acquired nasopharyngeal stenosis
Nasopharyngeal polyps
Polypoid rhinitis

Neoplasia

Adenocarcinoma, squamous cell carcinoma
Fibrosarcoma, osteosarcoma, chondrosarcoma
Lymphoma, transmissible venereal tumor, neuroendo-
  crine carcinoma

Foreign Body

Congenital

Cleft palate
Ciliary dyskinesia
Nasopharyngeal stenosis
Choanal atresia

Dental Disease

Tooth root abscess
Oronasal fistula

Trauma

Vascular Malformation

Systemic Disease

Infectious

Canine distemper virus
Canine infectious tracheobronchitis
Pneumonia

Hypertension

Hyperthyroidism
Hyperadrenocorticism
Renal disease
Pheochromocytoma
Hypothyroidism
Acromegaly
Polycythemia
Diabetes mellitus
Overhydration

Coagulopathies

Thrombocytopenia
Rocky Mountain spotted fever
Thrombocytopathia
von Willebrand disease
Factor deficiencies
Congenital (hemophilia A, B, others)
Acquired (vitamin K rodenticide toxicity, DIC, hepatic
failure)

Vasculitis

Toxic
Inflammatory
Immune mediated (SLE)
Neoplastic
Infectious (ehrlichiosis, FIP, Rocky Mountain spotted
fever, leishmaniasis)

Hyperviscosity

Multiple myeloma
Lymphoma
IgM (Waldenstrom) macroglobulinemia
Chronic lymphocytic leukemia
Ehrlichiosis
Amyloidosis
Plasma cell leukemia
FIP (rare)

Stertor and Stridor

Stertor

Snoring or snorting associated with partial nasal or nasopharyngeal obstruction.

Intranasal Disorders
    Congenital deformities
    Masses
    Exudates
    Clotted blood

Pharyngeal Disease
    Brachycephalic airway syndrome
    Elongated soft palate
    Nasopharyngeal polyp
    Foreign body
    Neoplasia
    Abscess
    Granuloma
    Extraluminal mass

Stridor

High-pitched wheeze caused by air turbulence in upper airway associated with laryngeal disease or narrowing of extrathoracic trachea.

Laryngeal Disease
    Neoplasia
    Polyps
    Laryngeal paralysis
    Laryngeal trauma
    Foreign body
    Acute laryngitis/obstructive laryngitis

Extrathoracic Tracheal Disease
    Neoplasia
    Foreign body
    Extrathoracic collapsing trachea
    Extraluminal mass

Stranguria, Dysuria, and Pollakiuria

Stranguria/Pollakiuria

Small Bladder
    Cystitis
    • Infectious agents
    • Idiopathic cystitis (cats)

Detrusor hyperspasticity
Urethritis
Urethral mass

Large Bladder
Lower urinary tract obstruction
- Functional
- Mechanical

Urinary Retention

Easy Catheterization
Normal Neurologic Examination
Cystic calculi or mass
Detrusor areflexia from overdistension
Reflex dyssynergia

Abnormal Neurologic Examination
Detrusor areflexia with sphincter areflexia (lower
motor neuron)
Detrusor areflexia with sphincter hypertonia (upper
motor neuron)
Dysautonomia

Difficult Catheterization
Urethral spasm
Urethral calculi
Urethral neoplasia
Transitional cell carcinoma
Granulomatous urethritis
Urethral inflammation
Prostatic disease
Mucoid or crystalline plug (cats)

Stomatitis

Infectious disease
- Feline immunodeficiency virus (FIV)
- Feline leukemia virus (FeLV)
- Feline syncytium-forming virus
- Feline calicivirus
- Feline herpesvirus
- Feline infectious peritonitis (FIP)
- Bartonellosis
- Canine distemper virus
- Feline panleukopenia virus
- Candidiasis
Immunosuppressive disease
Feline eosinophilic granuloma complex

Idiopathic feline chronic gingivitis/stomatitis
Immune-mediated disease
- Systemic lupus erythematosus (SLE)
- Bullous (pemphigus) disease
- Idiopathic vasculitis
- Toxic epidermal necrolysis
- Ulcerative gingivitis/stomatitis of Maltese Terriers
Uremic stomatitis
Radiation-induced

Stupor and Coma

Increased Intracranial Pressure

Encephalitis
Meningitis
Neoplasia
Granulomas
Abscess
Vascular events
Trauma
Underlying metabolic injury (e.g., hypertension)

Cerebral Edema

Vasogenic (brain masses that lead to breakdown of blood-
brain barrier)
Cytotoxic (hypoxia, neuroglycopenia)
Interstitial (hydrocephalus)

Herniation of Brain Tissue

Caudal transtentorial herniation
Foramen magnum herniation

Extracranial Causes

Hypoglycemia
Severe hypothyroidism
Toxins
Hepatic disease
Hyperadrenocorticism

Syncope

Normal Cerebral Perfusion

Severe hypoxemia
Hypoglycemia

Cerebral Hypoperfusion

Normotension
Cerebrovascular disease
Cerebral vasoconstriction

Systemic Hypotension
Decreased Cardiac Output
Loss of Preload
> Cardiac tamponade, atrial ball thrombi, atrial myxoma, atrioventricular (AV) valve stenosis, hypovolemia, diuretics

Obstruction to Flow
> Aortic and subaortic stenosis, pulmonic stenosis, pulmonary hypertension, pulmonary thromboembolism, outflow tract tumors, myocardial infarction, hypertropic and restrictive cardiomyopathy, systolic anterior motion of mitral valve, infundibular stenosis, heartworm disease

Arrhythmias
> Bradyarrhythmias: sick sinus syndrome, third-degree AV block, persistent atrial standstill, β-blockers, calcium channel blockers
> Tachyarrhythmias: atrial fibrillation, atrial tachycardia, AV reentrant tachycardia, ventricular tachycardia, drug-induced proarrhythmia, torsades de pointes

Loss of Vascular Resistance
> Drug therapy: angiotensin-converting enzyme (ACE) inhibitors, β-blockers, calcium channel blockers, hydralazine, nitrates, β-blockers, phenothiazines
> Reflex syncope (neurally mediated): orthostatic, postexertion, micturition, defecation, cough, emotional distress, pain, carotid sinus hypersensitivity
> Autonomic nervous system disease: primary or secondary (diabetes mellitus, paraneoplastic, chronic renal failure, autoimmune disease, amyloidosis)
> Cyanotic heart disease (tetralogy of Fallot, reversed shunt)

Tachycardia, Sinus

Anxiety/fear
Excitement
Exercise
Pain
Hyperthyroidism
Heart failure
Hyperthermia/fever
Anemia
Hypoxia
Shock
Hypotension
Sepsis
Drugs (anticholinergics, sympathomimetics)
Toxicity (e.g., chocolate, amphetamines, theophylline)
Electric shock
Any cause of high sympathetic tone

Tenesmus and Dyschezia

Colonic or Rectal Obstruction

Constipation Pelvic fracture
Rectal neoplasia
Extraluminal neoplasia
Prostatomegaly
Perineal hernia
Pelvic canal mass
Rectal granuloma
Rectal foreign body
Rectal stricture

Perineal Inflammation or Pain

Anal sacculitis
Perianal fistula
Perianal abscess/abscessed anal sac

Rectal Inflammation or Pain

Rectal tumor/polyp
Proctitis
Histoplasmosis
Pythiosis

Colonic Inflammation

Idiopathic colitis
Bacteria
Fungal

Parasites
Dietary indiscretion
Inflammatory bowel disease
Neoplasia

Tremor

Physiologic Tremor

Hypothermia
Heavy exercise/exhaustion

Pathologic Tremor

Metabolic disorders (renal disease, hypoglycemia,
hypocalcemia, hypoadrenocorticism)
Intracranial infectious disease (*Neospora caninum,* cerebellar
hypoplasia secondary to intrauterine panleukopenia infection)
Intracranial disease (fibrinoid leukodystrophy, neuraxonal
dystrophy, Labrador Retriever axonopathy, spongiform
encephalopathy, neuronal abiotrophies, subacute
necrotizing encephalopathy, lysosomal storage diseases)
Hind end tremor (intervertebral disk herniation, tumors,
diskospondylitis, nerve root compression, peripheral
neuropathies)
Corticoid-responsive tremor syndrome (formerly "white
shaker disease")
Myasthenia gravis
Cerebellar malformation
Hypomyelination
Spongy degeneration
Tremorgenic toxins (mycotoxins penitrem A and
roquefortine produced by *Penicillium* spp. growing
on spoiled foods; metaldehyde, hexachlorophene,
bromethalin, organophosphates, carbamates, pyrethroids,
xanthines, macadamia nuts, strychnine)
Idiopathic head tremor in Doberman Pinschers and Bulldogs
Idiopathic tremor of hind legs of geriatric dogs

Urine, Discolored

Red, Pink, Red-Brown, Red-Orange, or Orange

Hematuria
Hemoglobinuria
Myoglobinuria
Porphyrinuria
Pyuria

Orange-Yellow

Highly concentrated urine
Urobilin
Bilirubin

Yellow-Brown or Green-Brown

Bile pigments

Brown to Black

Melanin
Methemoglobin
Myoglobin
Bile pigments

Brown

Methemoglobin
Melanin

Colorless

Dilute urine

Milky White

Lipid
Pyuria
Crystals

Pale Yellow

Normal
Dilute urine

Urticaria/Angioedema

Immediate Hypersensitivity Reaction

Insect bites/stings
Food
Drugs/vaccines
Airborne allergens (atopy)

Nonimmunologic Stimulus by Irritant

Weeds
Insects
Physical stimuli (cold, heat, sunlight)
Psychogenic stimuli

Vision Loss, Sudden

See **Blindness.**

Vomiting

Gastric Disease

Gastritis
Parasites
Foreign body
Obstruction
Ulceration
Neoplasia
Dilatation/volvulus
Helicobacter infection
Gastric ulcer
Hiatal hernia
Motility disorders
Pyloric stenosis
Gastric antral mucosal hypertrophy

Small Intestinal Disease

Parasites
Inflammatory bowel disease
Foreign body
Bacterial overgrowth/enteritis
Hemorrhagic gastroenteritis
Neoplasia
Viral enteritis (parvovirus, canine distemper virus)
Intussusception
Nonneoplastic infiltrative disease (e.g., pythiosis)

Large Intestinal Disease

Colitis
Obstipation
Parasites

Dietary

Indiscretion
Intolerance
Allergy

Drugs

Cancer chemotherapeutic agents
Antibiotics (especially erythromycin, tetracycline)
Nonsteroidal antiinflammatory drugs (NSAIDs)
Cardiac glycosides
Apomorphine
Xylazine
Penicillamine

Extraalimentary Tract Disease

Peritonitis
Pancreatitis
Hepatobiliary disease
Neoplasia
Uremia
Diabetes mellitus/ketoacidosis
Hyperthyroidism
Hypoadrenocorticism
Hepatic disease
Hepatic encephalopathy
Septicemia/endotoxemia
Pyometra
Acid-base disorders
Electrolyte disorders
Hypertriglyceridemia
Gastrinoma (Zollinger-Ellison syndrome)
Mastocytosis

Intoxicants

Numerous inorganic, organic, and plant toxins can cause gastro-intestinal irritation and vomiting.

Neurologic Disease

Epilepsy, tumor, meningitis, increased intracranial pressure, dysautonomia

Weakness

Very nonspecific clinical sign of disease
Metabolic disease
Inflammation
- Infectious disease (bacterial, viral, fungal, rickettsial, protozoal, parasitic)
- Immune-mediated disease
Fever
Electrolyte disorders
- Hypokalemia, hyperkalemia, hyponatremia, hypernatremia, hypocalcemia, hypomagnesemia
Acid-base disorders
Anemia
Poor oxygen delivery

Endocrine disease
* Diabetes mellitus, hypothyroidism, hypoadrenocorticism, hyperadrenocorticism, hypoglycemia, hyperparathyroidism, hypoparathyroidism, pheochromocytoma

Cardiovascular disease

Hypotension, hypertension

Respiratory disease

Neuromuscular disease
* Brain disease (encephalitis, cerebrovascular accidents, space-occupying lesions, vestibular disease, idiopathic epilepsy)
* Spinal cord diseases
* Neuropathies (e.g., polyradiculoneuritis, myasthenia gravis, developmental disorders, toxoplasmosis, neosporosis)

Neoplasia

Cachexia

Physical and psychologic stress

Malnutrition

Drugs
* Anticonvulsants, antihistamines, glucocorticoids, tranquilizers, narcotics, cardiac drugs

Toxins

Pain

Weight Gain

See **Obesity.**

Weight Loss

See **Cachexia and Muscle Wasting.**

Systemic Approach to Differential Diagnosis

Cardiopulmonary Disorders

Arrhythmias

Differential Diagnosis

Slow, Irregular Rhythms
Sinus bradyarrhythmias
Sinus arrest
Sick sinus syndrome
High-grade second-degree atrioventricular (AV) block

Slow, Regular Rhythms
Sinus bradycardia
Complete AV block with ventricular escape rhythm
Atrial standstill with ventricular escape rhythm

Fast, Irregular Rhythms
Atrial or supraventricular premature contractions
Paroxysmal atrial or supraventricular tachycardia
Atrial flutter

Atrial fibrillation
Ventricular premature contractions
Paroxysmal ventricular tachycardia

Fast, Regular Rhythms
Sinus tachycardia
Sustained supraventricular tachycardia
Sustained ventricular tachycardia

Normal, Irregular Rhythms (require no treatment)
Respiratory sinus arrhythmia
Wandering pacemaker

Arterial Thromboembolism

Clinical Findings

Acute Limb Paresis
Posterior paresis ("saddle" thrombus: most common presentation)
Monoparesis (right subclavian artery thrombus; second most common presentation in cats)
Intermittent claudication
Severe limb pain
Cool distal limbs
Cyanotic nail beds
Arterial pulse absent
Contracture of affected muscles
Vocalization (pain, distress)

Renal Infarction
Renal pain
Acute renal failure

Splenic Infarction
Lethargy
Anorexia
Vomiting
Diarrhea

Mesenteric Infarction
Abdominal pain
Vomiting
Diarrhea

Cerebral Infarction
Neurologic deficits
Seizures
Sudden death

Signs of Heart Failure
Systolic murmur
Gallop rhythm
Tachypnea/dyspnea
Weakness/lethargy
Anorexia
Arrhythmias
Hypothermia
Cardiomegaly
Effusions
Pulmonary edema

Hematologic and Biochemical Abnormalities
Azotemia
Increased alanine aminotransferase activity
Increased aspartate aminotransferase activity
Increased lactate dehydrogenase activity
Increased creatine kinase activity
Hyperglycemia
Lymphopenia
Disseminated intravascular coagulation

Aspiration Pneumonia

Etiology of Aspiration Pneumonia

Esophageal Disorders
Megaesophagus
Reflux esophagitis
Esophageal obstruction
Myasthenia gravis (localized)
Bronchoesophageal fistulae

Localized Oropharyngeal Disorders
Cleft palate
Cricopharyngeal motor dysfunction
Laryngoplasty
Brachycephalic airway syndrome

Systemic Neuromuscular Disorders
Myasthenia gravis
Polyneuropathy
Polymyopathy

Decreased Mentation
General anesthesia
Sedation
Post ictus

Head trauma
Severe metabolic disease

Iatrogenic
Force-feeding
Stomach tubes

Vomiting (in combination with other predisposing factors)

Atrioventricular Valve Disease, Chronic (Mitral or Tricuspid Valve)

Potential Complications

Acute Worsening of Pulmonary Edema
Arrhythmias
- Frequent atrial premature contractions
- Paroxysmal atrial/supraventricular contractions
- Atrial fibrillation
- Ventricular tachyarrhythmias

Ruptured chordae tendineae
Iatrogenic volume overload
- Excessive fluid or blood administration
- High-sodium fluids

High sodium intake
Increased cardiac workload
- Physical exertion
- Anemia
- Infection/sepsis
- Hypertension
- Disease of other organ systems (pulmonary, hepatic, renal, endocrine)
- Environmental stress (heat, humidity, cold, etc.)

Inadequate medication for stage of disease
Erratic or improper drug administration
Myocardial degeneration and poor contractility

Causes of Reduced Cardiac Output
Arrhythmias
Ruptured chordae tendineae
Cough-related syncope
Left atrial tear, intrapericardial bleeding, cardiac tamponade
Secondary right-sided heart failure
Myocardial degeneration, poor contractility

Cardiomegaly

Differential Diagnosis

Generalized Cardiomegaly
Dilated cardiomyopathy
Pericardial effusion
Mitral and tricuspid valve insufficiency
Tricuspid dysplasia
Pericardioperitoneal diaphragmatic hernia
Ventricular septal defect
Patent ductus arteriosus

Left Atrial Enlargement
Mitral valve insufficiency
Hypertrophic cardiomyopathy
Early dilated cardiomyopathy (especially in Doberman
  Pinschers)
Subaortic or aortic stenosis

Left Atrial and Ventricular Enlargement
Dilated cardiomyopathy
Hypertrophic cardiomyopathy
Mitral valve insufficiency
Aortic valve insufficiency
Ventricular septal defect
Patent ductus arteriosus
Subaortic or aortic stenosis
Systemic hypertension
Hyperthyroidism

Right Atrial and Ventricular Enlargement
Advanced heartworm disease
Chronic severe pulmonary disease
Tricuspid valve insufficiency
Atrial septal defect
Pulmonic stenosis
Tetralogy of Fallot
Reversed-shunting congenital defects
Pulmonary hypertension
Mass lesion within right heart

Chylothorax

Diagnostic Criteria

Protein concentration is greater than 2.5 g/dL
Nucleated cell count ranges from 400 to 10,000/μL

Predominant cell type on cytology is the small lymphocyte
(also see neutrophils, macrophages, plasma cells, and
mesothelial cells)

Triglyceride concentration of pleural fluid is greater than
that of serum (definitive test)

Causes of Chylothorax

Traumatic
* Blunt force trauma (e.g., vehicular trauma)
* Postthoracotomy

Nontraumatic
* Neoplasia (especially mediastinal lymphoma in cats)
* Cardiomyopathy
* Dirofilariasis
* Pericardial disease
* Other causes of right heart failure
* Lung lobe torsion
* Diaphragmatic hernia
* Systemic lymphangiectasia

Idiopathic (most commonly diagnosed)

Diagnostic Tests to Identify Underlying Cause of Chylothorax in Dogs and Cats

CBC, Serum Chemistry, Urinalysis
* Evaluation of systemic status

Cytologic Examination of Pleural Fluid
* Infectious agents
* Neoplastic cells

Thoracic Radiographs (after fluid removal)
* Cranial mediastinal masses
* Other neoplasia
* Cardiac disease
* Heartworm disease
* Pericardial disease

Ultrasonography (before fluid removal)
* Cranial mediastinum (masses)
* Echocardiography (cardiomyopathy, heartworm disease,
  pericardial disease, congenital heart disease)
* Ultrasound of body wall and pleural space (neoplasia,
  lung lobe torsion)

Heartworm Antibody and Antigen Tests
* Heartworm disease

Lymphangiography
- Preoperative and postoperative assessment of thoracic duct

Congenital Heart Disease

Breed Predispositions

Patent Ductus Arteriosus
Maltese, Pomeranian, Shetland Sheepdog, English Cocker Spaniel, English Springer Spaniel, Keeshond, Bichon Frise, toy and miniature Poodle, Yorkshire Terrier, Collie, Cocker Spaniel, German Shepherd, Chihuahua, Kerry Blue Terrier, Labrador Retriever, Newfoundland; female affected more than male

Subaortic Stenosis
Newfoundland, Golden Retriever, Rottweiler, Boxer, German Shepherd, English Bulldog, Great Dane, German Shorthaired Pointer, Bouvier des Flandres, Samoyed

Aortic Stenosis
Bull Terrier

Pulmonic Stenosis
English Bulldog (male affected more than female), Mastiff, Samoyed, Miniature Schnauzer, Newfoundland, West Highland White Terrier, Cocker Spaniel, Beagle, Basset Hound, Airedale Terrier, Boykin Spaniel, Chihuahua, Scottish Terrier, Boxer, Fox Terrier, Chow Chow, Labrador Retriever, Schnauzer

Atrial Septal Defect
Samoyed, Doberman Pinscher, Boxer

Ventricular Septal Defect
English Bulldog, English Springer Spaniel, Keeshond, West Highland White Terrier, cats

Tricuspid Dysplasia
Labrador Retriever, German Shepherd, Boxer, Weimaraner, Great Dane, Old English Sheepdog, Golden Retriever, various other large breeds

Mitral Dysplasia
Bull Terrier, German Shepherd, Great Dane, Golden Retriever, Newfoundland, Mastiff, Rottweiler, cats

Tetralogy of Fallot
Keeshond, English Bulldog

Persistent Right Aortic Arch
German Shepherd, Great Dane, Irish Setter

Cor Triatriatum
Medium- to large-breed dogs (Chow Chow), rarely small-breed dogs or cats

Peritoneopericardial Diaphragmatic Hernia
Weimaraner

Heart Failure

Causes of Chronic Heart Failure

Left-Sided Heart Failure

Volume-Flow Overload
Mitral valve regurgitation (degenerative, congenital, infective)
Aortic regurgitation (infective endocardiosis, congenital)
Ventricular septal defect
Patent ductus arteriosis

Myocardial Failure
Myocardial ischemia/infarction
Drug toxicity (e.g., doxorubicin)

Pressure Overload
Aortic/subaortic stenosis
Systemic hypertension

Restriction of Ventricular Filling
Hypertrophic cardiomyopathy
Restrictive cardiomyopathy

Left- or Right-Sided Heart Failure

Myocardial Failure
Idiopathic dilated cardiomyopathy
Infective myocarditis

Volume-Flow Overload
Chronic anemia
Thyrotoxicosis

Right-Sided Heart Failure

Volume-Flow Overload
Tricuspid endocarditis
Tricuspid endocardiosis
Tricuspid dysplasia

Pressure Overload
Pulmonic stenosis
Heartworm disease
Pulmonary hypertension

Restriction to Ventricular Filling
  Cardiac tamponade
  Constrictive pericardial disease

Severity

Classification Systems

New York Heart Association Functional Classification

Class I: Heart disease present, but no evidence of heart failure or exercise intolerance; cardiomegaly minimal to absent

Class II: Signs of heart disease with evidence of exercise intolerance; radiographic cardiomegaly present

Class III: Signs of heart failure with normal activity or signs at night (e.g., cough, orthopnea); radiographic signs of significant cardiomegaly and pulmonary edema or pleural/abdominal effusion

Class IV: Severe heart failure with clinical signs at rest or with minimal activity; marked radiographic signs of congestive heart failure (CHF) and cardiomegaly

Forrester Classification

Class I: Normal cardiac output and pulmonary venous pressure

Class II: Pulmonary congestion but normal cardiac output

Class III: Low cardiac output and peripheral hypoperfusion with no pulmonary congestion

Class IV: Low cardiac output with pulmonary congestion

Clinical Findings

Low-Output Signs
  Exercise intolerance
  Syncope
  Weak arterial pulses
  Tachycardia
  Arrhythmias
  Cold extremities
  Prerenal azotemia
  Cyanosis

Signs Related to Poor Skeletal Muscle Function
  Weight loss
  Exercise intolerance

Dyspnea
Decreased muscle mass

Signs Related to Fluid Retention

Left-Sided Heart Failure (Pulmonary Edema)

Dyspnea/orthopnea
Exercise intolerance
Wet lung sounds
Tachypnea
Gallop rhythm
Functional mitral regurgitation
Cyanosis
Cough

Right-Sided Heart Failure

Ascites
Subcutaneous edema
Jugular distension/pulsation
Hepatomegaly
Splenomegaly
Hepatojugular reflux
Gallop rhythm
Cardiac arrhythmias

Bilateral Signs

Pleural effusion (dyspnea, muffled heart sounds, cough)

Heartworm Disease

Clinical Findings

Historical Findings

Asymptomatic
Cough
Dyspnea
Weight loss
Lethargy
Exercise intolerance
Poor condition
Syncope
Abdominal distension (ascites)

Physical Findings

Weight loss
Right-sided murmur (tricuspid insufficiency)
Split-second heart sound
Gallop rhythm
Cough

Pulmonary crackles
Dyspnea
Muffled breath sounds
Cyanosis
Right-sided heart failure
- Jugular distension/pulsation
- Hepatosplenomegaly
- Ascites
Pulmonary thromboembolism
- Dyspnea/tachypnea
- Fever
- Hemoptysis
Cardiac arrhythmias/conduction disturbances (rare)
Caval syndrome
- Hemoglobinuria
- Anemia
- Disseminated intravascular coagulation (DIC)
- Icterus
- Collapse/death

Clinicopathologic Findings

Eosinophilia
Nonregenerative anemia
Neutrophilia
Basophilia
Proteinuria
Hyperbilirubinemia
Azotemia
Thrombocytopenia

Radiographic Signs

Right ventricular enlargement
Prominent main pulmonary artery segment
Increased pulmonary artery size
Tortuous pulmonary vessels
Caudal vena cava enlargement
Hepatosplenomegaly
Ascites
Pleural effusion
Bronchial/interstitial lung disease

Diagnosis in Dogs

Antigen Test Positive and Modified Knott's or Filter Test Negative

- Perform complete blood count, serum chemistry panel, urinalysis, thoracic radiography
- Start preventative and adulticidal therapy

- Antigen test positive and Modified Knott's or filter test positive
- Perform complete blood count, serum chemistry panel, urinalysis, and thoracic radiography
- Start "slow kill" macrolide and adulticidal therapy

Antigen Test Negative
- No infection or low heartworm burden
- Start preventative

Hypertension

Pulmonary Hypertension

Potential Clinical Signs
Ascites
Jugular venous distension/pulsation
Subcutaneous edema
Cachexia
Nonspecific respiratory signs
- Coughing
- Tachypnea
- Respiratory distress
- Increased bronchovesicular sounds
- Hemoptysis

Cyanosis
- Right-to-left cardiac shunts
- Severe respiratory disease

Split or loud pulmonic component to second heart sound
Right or left apical systolic murmurs (tricuspid or mitral regurgitation)

Radiographic Signs
Cardiomegaly
Right ventricular enlargement
Dilated central pulmonary arteries with tapering toward periphery
Eisenmenger complex (pulmonary undercirculation and right-sided heart enlargement)
Left atrial enlargement and perihilar to caudodorsal pulmonary infiltrates (left-sided congestive heart failure)

Echocardiographic Signs
Right ventricular concentric hypertrophy and dilation
Main pulmonary artery and main branch dilation
Systolic flattening of interventricular septum

Paradoxical septal motion
Reduced left ventricular dimensions in severe pulmonary
hypertension caused by ventricular underfilling

Laboratory Values
Acidosis
Rule out heartworm disease

Systemic Hypertension

Causes of Systemic Hypertension in Dogs and Cats
Renal failure (chronic or acute)
Hyperadrenocorticism
Diabetes mellitus
Pheochromocytoma
Hyperthyroidism
Liver disease
Hyperaldosteronism
Intracranial lesions (↑ intracranial pressure)
High-salt diet
Obesity
Chronic anemia (cats)

Clinical Signs of Systemic Hypertension
Ocular Findings
Hypertensive choroidopathy (edema, vascular
tortuosity, hemorrhage, focal ischemia)
Hypertensive retinopathy (edema, vascular tortuosity,
hemorrhage, focal ischemia, atrophy)
Intraocular hemorrhage (retinal, vitreal, hyphema)
Papilledema
Blindness
Glaucoma
Secondary corneal ulcers

Neurologic Findings
Edema (↑ intracranial pressure)
Hypertensive encephalopathy (lethargy, behavioral
changes)
Cerebrovascular accident (focal ischemia, hemorrhage)
Seizures/collapse

Renal
Polyuria/polydipsia
Glomerulosclerosis/proliferative glomerulitis
Renal tubular degenerative and fibrosis
Further deterioration in renal function

Cardiac
Left ventricular hypertrophy
Murmur or gallop sound
Aortic dilation
Aneurysm or dissection rare

Other
Epistaxis

Laryngeal and Pharyngeal Disease

Differential Diagnosis

Laryngeal paralysis
Brachycephalic airway syndrome
Acute laryngitis
Laryngeal neoplasia
Nasopharyngeal polyp
Abscess
Tonsillitis
Pharyngitis
Obstructive laryngitis
Laryngeal collapse
Trauma
Foreign body
Extraluminal mass
Elongated soft palate
Cleft palate
Soft palate hypoplasia
Pharyngeal neoplasia
Granuloma
Pharyngeal mucoceles
Web formation
Nasopharyngeal stenosis

Causes of Laryngeal Paralysis

Idiopathic

Polyneuropathy and Polymyopathy
Idiopathic
Immune-mediated
Endocrinopathy
- Hypothyroidism
- Hypoadrenocorticism
Toxicity
Congenital disease

Ventral Cervical Lesion

Nerve trauma
- Direct trauma
- Inflammation
- Fibrosis

Neoplasia
Other inflammatory or mass lesion

Anterior Thoracic Lesion

Neoplasia
Trauma
- Postoperative
- Other

Other inflammatory or mass lesion

Myasthenia Gravis

Lower Respiratory Tract Disease

Differential Diagnosis

Disorders of Trachea and Bronchi

Canine infectious tracheobronchitis
Collapsing trachea
Bacterial infection
Mycoplasmal infection
Bronchial asthma
Neoplasia
Allergic bronchitis
Feline bronchitis
Bronchial compression
- Left atrial enlargement
- Hilar lymphadenopathy

Acute bronchitis
Canine chronic bronchitis/bronchiectasis
Parasites *(Oslerus osleri, Filaroides osleri)*
Tracheal tear
Primary ciliary dyskinesia
Airway foreign body
Chronic aspiration

Disorders of Pulmonary Parenchyma

Infectious disease
- Viral pneumonia (canine influenza, canine distemper virus, canine adenovirus, canine parainfluenza, feline calicivirus, feline infectious peritonitis, pneumonia secondary to feline leukemia virus or feline immunodeficiency virus)

- Bacterial pneumonia
- Protozoal pneumonia (toxoplasmosis)
- Fungal pneumonia (blastomycosis, histoplasmosis, coccidioidomycosis)
- Rickettsial disease (*Rickettsia rickettsii, Ehrlichia* spp.)
- Parasitism
  - Heartworm disease
  - Pulmonary parasites (*Paragonimus, Aelurostrongylus, Capillaria, Crenosoma* spp.)
  - Larval migration of *Toxocara canis*

Aspiration pneumonia
Pulmonary infiltrates with eosinophils
Eosinophilic pulmonary granulomatosis
Aspiration pneumonia
Pulmonary neoplasia (primary, metastatic, lymphosarcoma, lymphomatoid granulomatosis, malignant histiocytosis)
Pulmonary hypertension
Pulmonary contusions
Pulmonary thromboembolism
Pulmonary edema
Acute respiratory distress syndrome
Lung lobe torsion
Pulmonary fibrosis
Pickwickian syndrome (obesity)
Idiopathic interstitial pneumonias

Mediastinal Disease

Differential Diagnosis of Lesions Associated with Focal Mediastinal Enlargement

Pneumomediastinum
Mediastinitis (*Histoplasma, Cryptococcus, Actinomyces, Nocardia, Spirocerca* spp.)
Mediastinal hemorrhage
Mediastinal cysts
Nonneoplastic mediastinal masses (fungal pyogranulomas, abscesses, granulomas, lymphadenopathy, hematomas)
Mediastinal neoplasia (lymphosarcoma)
Thymoma
Obesity
Thymic hemorrhage
Heart base mass
Neurogenic tumor
Tracheal mass
Esophageal mass, foreign body, or dilatation

Ectopic thyroid tissue
Mediastinal edema
Vascular mass (aorta, cranial vena cava)
Paraspinal or spinal mass
Aortic stenosis
Patent ductus arteriosus
Left atrial enlargement
Main pulmonary artery mass (poststenotic dilatation)
Hiatal hernia
Diaphragmatic hernia or mass
Aortic aneurysm
Gastroesophageal intussusception
Peritoneopericardial diaphragmatic hernia

Myocardial Diseases

Differential Diagnosis, Dogs

Dilated Cardiomyopathy

Primary (idiopathic, most common)

Genetic (Doberman Pinscher, Boxer, Cocker Spaniel, Great Dane, Portuguese Water Dog, Newfoundland, Dalmatian, Irish Wolfhound)

Secondary

Nutritional Deficiencies

L-Carnitine (Boxer, Doberman Pinscher, Great Dane, Irish Wolfhound, Newfoundland, Cocker Spaniel)
Taurine

Myocardial Infection

Viral myocarditis (acute viral infections, e.g., parvovirus)
Bacterial myocarditis (secondary to bacteremia from infections elsewhere in body)
Lyme disease: *Borrelia burgdorferi*
Protozoal myocarditis *(Trypanosoma cruzi [Chagas disease], Toxoplasma gondii, Neospora caninum, Babesia canis, Hepatozoon canis)*
Fungal myocarditis (rare, *Aspergillus, Cryptococcus, Coccidioides, Histoplasma, Paecilomyces* spp.)
Rickettsial myocarditis (rare, *Rickettsia rickettsii, Ehrlichia canis, Bartonella* spp.)
Algae-like organisms (rare, *Prototheca* spp.)
Nematode larval migration (*Toxocara* spp.)

Trauma

Ischemia

Infiltrative Neoplasia

Hyperthermia

Irradiation

Electric Shock

Cardiotoxins
Doxorubicin; ethyl alcohol; plant toxins such as foxglove, black locust, buttercup, lily of the valley, and gossypol; cocaine; anesthetic drugs; catecholamines; monensin

Hypertrophic Cardiomyopathy (uncommon in dogs)

Arrhythmogenic Right Ventricular Cardiomyopathy (rare)

Noninfective Myocarditis
Catecholamines; heavy metals; antineoplastic drugs (doxorubicin, cyclophosphamide, 5-fluorouracil, interleukin-2, interferon-α); stimulant drugs (thyroid hormone, cocaine, amphetamines, lithium)
Immune-mediated diseases, pheochromocytoma
Wasp and scorpion stings, snake venom, spider bite

Differential Diagnosis, Cats

Hypertrophic Cardiomyopathy
Primary (Idiopathic)
Maine Coon, Persian, Ragdoll, and American shorthair may be predisposed.

Secondary
Hyperthyroidism
Hypersomatotropism (acromegaly)
Infiltrative myocardial disease (lymphoma)

Restrictive Cardiomyopathy

Dilated Cardiomyopathy
Taurine-deficient diets
Doxorubicin
End stage of other myocardial metabolic, toxic, or infectious process

Arrhythmogenic Right Ventricular Cardiomyopathy

Myocarditis
Viral (coronavirus, other viruses)

Bacterial (bacteremia, *Bartonella* spp.)
Protozoal *(Toxoplasma gondii)*

Murmurs

Clinical Findings

Systolic Murmurs

Functional murmurs (point of maximal impulse
[PMI] over left-sided heart base, decrescendo or
crescendo-decrescendo)
- Innocent puppy murmurs
- Physiologic murmurs (anemia, fever, high sympathetic
  tone, hyperthyroidism, peripheral arteriovenous
  fistula, marked bradycardia, hypoproteinemia, athletic
  heart)

Mitral valve insufficiency (left apex, typically
holosystolic)

Ejection murmurs (typically left-sided heart base)
- Subaortic stenosis (low left base and right base)
- Pulmonic stenosis (high left base)
- Dynamic muscular obstruction

Right-sided murmurs (usually holosystolic)
- Tricuspid insufficiency (right apex, may see jugular
  pulse)
- Ventricular septal defect (PMI over right sternal
  border)

Diastolic Murmurs

Aortic insufficiency from bacterial endocarditis (left-sided
heart base)
Aortic valve congenital malformations (left base)
Aortic valve degenerative disease (left base)
Pulmonic insufficiency (left base)

Continuous Murmurs

Patent ductus arteriosus (PMI high left base above
pulmonic area)

Concurrent Systolic and Diastolic Murmurs
(To-and-Fro Murmurs)

Subaortic stenosis with aortic insufficiency
Pulmonic stenosis with pulmonic insufficiency

Grading

Grade I: Very soft murmur; heard only in quiet
surroundings after minutes of listening

Grade II: Soft murmur but easily heard
Grade III: Moderate-intensity murmur
Grade IV: Loud murmur; no precordial thrill
Grade V: Loud murmur with palpable precordial thrill
Grade VI: Very loud murmur; can be heard with
  stethoscope off chest wall; palpable precordial thrill

Pericardial Effusion

Differential Diagnosis

Bacterial Pericarditis
  Secondary to foxtail (*Hordeum* spp.) migration
  Secondary to penetrating animal bite
  Disseminated tuberculosis

Fungal Pericarditis
  Coccidioidomycosis
  Aspergillosis
  Actinomycosis

Viral Pericarditis
  Feline infectious peritonitis (FIP)
  Canine distemper virus

Protozoal Pericarditis
  Toxoplasmosis
  Other systemic protozoal infections

Left Atrial Rupture (Secondary to Mitral Valve Disease)

Neoplasia
  Hemangiosarcoma
  Mesothelioma
  Heart base tumor (aortic body tumor or chemodectoma,
    ectopic thyroid tumor, ectopic parathyroid tumor,
    connective tissue neoplasms)
  Lymphosarcoma
  Rhabdomyosarcoma

Other
  Penetrating trauma
  Pericardioperitoneal diaphragmatic hernia
  Hypoalbuminemia
  Pericardial cyst
  Coagulation disorders
  Congestive heart failure
  Uremia
  Idiopathic

Pleural Effusion

Differential Diagnosis

Transudates and Modified Transudates
Right-sided heart failure
Pericardial disease
Hypoalbuminemia
Neoplasia
Diaphragmatic hernia

Nonseptic Exudates
Feline infectious peritonitis (FIP)
Neoplasia
Diaphragmatic hernia
Lung lobe torsion

Septic Exudates
Pyothorax

Chylous Effusion
Chylothorax

Hemorrhage
Trauma
Bleeding disorder
Neoplasia
Lung lobe torsion

Diagnostic Approach in Dogs and Cats with Pleural Effusion Based on Fluid Type

Pure and Modified Transudates
Right-sided heart failure, pericardial effusion (evaluate pulses, auscultation, ECG, thoracic radiography, echocardiography)
Hypoalbuminemia (serum albumin concentration)
Neoplasia, diaphragmatic hernia (thoracic radiography, thoracic ultrasound, CT, thoracoscopy, thoracotomy)

Nonseptic Exudates
Feline infectious peritonitis (pleural fluid cytology [most reliable test], CBC, serum chemistry, ophthalmoscopic examination, serum or fluid electrophoresis, coronavirus antibody titer, PCR of tissues or effusion)
Neoplasia, diaphragmatic hernia (thoracic radiography, thoracic ultrasound, CT, thoracoscopy, thoracotomy)
Lung lobe torsion (thoracic radiography, ultrasound, bronchoscopy, thoracotomy)

Septic Exudates
Pyothorax (Gram stain, aerobic and anaerobic culture, cytology)

Chylous Effusion
Chylothorax (protein concentration, nucleated cell count, cytology, triglyceride)

Hemorrhagic
Trauma (history)

Bleeding disorder (systemic examination, coagulation tests platelet count)

Neoplasia (thoracic radiography, thoracic ultrasound, CT, thoracoscopy, thoracotomy)

Lung lobe torsion (thoracic radiography, ultrasound, bronchoscopy, thoracotomy)

Pulmonary Disease

Differential Diagnosis Based on Radiographic Patterns

Alveolar Pattern
Pulmonary edema (cardiogenic or noncardiogenic)

Infectious pneumonia (bacterial, parasitic, protozoal, viral)

Aspiration pneumonia

Atelectasis

Drowning

Smoke inhalation

Hemorrhage
- Neoplasia (primary and metastatic)
- Fungal pneumonia (severe)
- Pulmonary contusion
- Thromboembolic disease
- Systemic coagulopathy

Bronchial Pattern
Feline bronchitis/asthma

Allergic bronchitis

Bacterial bronchitis

Canine chronic bronchitis

Bronchiectasis

Pulmonary parasites

Bronchial calcification

Vascular Pattern
Enlarged Arteries
Heartworm disease

Thromboembolic disease
Pulmonary hypertension

Enlarged Veins
Left-sided heart failure

Enlarged Arteries and Veins (Pulmonary Overcirculation)

Left-to-Right Shunts
Patent ductus arteriosus
Ventricular septal defect
Atrial septal defect

Small Arteries and Veins
Pulmonary Undercirculation
Cardiovascular shock
Hypovolemia
- Severe dehydration
- Blood loss
- Hypoadrenocorticism
Pulmonic valve stenosis

Hyperinflation of Lungs
Feline bronchitis
Allergic bronchitis

Nodular Interstitial Pattern
Mycotic infection
- Blastomycosis
- Histoplasmosis
- Coccidioidomycosis
Neoplasia
Pulmonary parasites
- Aelurostrongylus infection
- Paragonimus infection
Pulmonary abscess
- Bacterial pneumonia
- Foreign body
Pulmonary infiltrates with eosinophils
Miscellaneous inflammatory diseases
Inactive lesions

Reticular Interstitial Patterns
Infection
- Viral pneumonia
- Bacterial pneumonia
- Toxoplasmosis
- Mycotic pneumonia
Parasitic infestation
Neoplasia

Pulmonary fibrosis
Pulmonary infiltrates with eosinophils
Miscellaneous inflammatory diseases
Hemorrhage (mild)
Old dog lung

Pulmonary Edema

Causes

Vascular Overload

Cardiogenic
- Left-sided heart murmur
- Left-to-right shunt

Overhydration

Decreased Plasma Oncotic Pressure

Hypoalbuminemia
- Gastrointestinal loss
- Renal loss (glomerular disease)
- Liver disease (lack of production)
- Iatrogenic overhydration

Increased Vascular Permeability

Sepsis
Shock
Drugs or toxins
Snake envenomation
Cisplatin (cats)
Trauma
- Pulmonary
- Multisystemic

Inhaled toxins
- Smoke inhalation
- Gastric acid aspiration
- Oxygen toxicity

Electrocution
Pancreatitis
Uremia
Virulent babesiosis
Disseminated intravascular coagulation
Inflammation/Vasculitis

Other Causes

Thromboembolism
Postobstruction (strangulation, laryngeal paralysis,
   pulmonary reexpansion)
Near-drowning

Neurogenic edema
- Seizures
- Head trauma

Lung lobe torsion
Bacterial pneumonia
Pulmonary contusion
Hyperoxia
High altitude
Air embolus
Pheochromocytoma

Lymphatic Obstruction (rare)

Neoplasia

Pulmonary Thromboembolism

Causes

Embolization of Thrombi (any condition that predisposes to venous stasis, endothelial injury, and hypercoagulability)

Heartworm disease
Immune-mediated hemolytic anemia
Systemic inflammatory disease
Neoplasia
Cardiac disease
Cardiomyopathy
Endocarditis
Congestive heart failure
Protein-losing nephropathy
Protein-losing enteropathy
Hyperadrenocorticism
Pancreatitis
Disseminated intravascular coagulation
Anatomic abnormality (e.g., aneurysm, A-V fistula)
Hyperviscosity (polycythemia, leukemia, hyperglobulinemia)
Hypoviscosity (anemia)
Sepsis
Shock
Intravenous catheterization
Injection of irritating substance
Prolonged recumbency
Reperfusion injury
Atherosclerosis/Arteriosclerosis
Trauma
Recent surgery
Hyperhomocysteinemia

Embolization of Parasites
Heartworm disease

Embolization of Fat

Embolization of Neoplastic Cells

Tachycardia, Sinus

Causes

Anxiety/fear
Excitement
Exercise
Pain
Hyperthyroidism
Hyperthermia/fever
Anemia
Hypoxia
Shock
Hypotension
Sepsis
Drugs (anticholinergics, sympathomimetics)
Toxicity (e.g., chocolate, hexachlorophene)
Electric shock

Dermatologic Disorders

Allergic Skin Disease

Clinical Findings

Flea Allergy

Dogs

Papular rash
Caudal distribution of lesions most common

Cats

Miliary dermatitis, especially over caudal back, around neck and chin
Eosinophilic granuloma complex

Atopy and Cutaneous Signs of Food Hypersensitivity

Signs of these two types of allergy are similar.
Atopy tends to occur primarily in young adults, whereas food hypersensitivity can begin at any age. Atopy is usually seasonal at first but may become less seasonal.

Dogs

Papular rash
Pruritus and self-trauma
Lesions of face, ears, feet, and perineum
Recurrent otitis externa
Excoriation
Lichenification
Pigmentary changes
Secondary pyoderma

Cats

Miliary dermatitis
Eosinophilic dermatitis

Allergic Contact Dermatitis

Rarest of allergic dermatoses

Lesions tend to be confined to hairless or sparsely haired skin (ventral abdomen, neck, and chest; ventral paws but not pads; perineum; lateral aspect of pinnae).

Acutely: Erythema, macules, papules, vesicles

Chronically: Alopecic plaques, hyperpigmentation, hypopigmentation, excoriation, lichenification

Alopecia, Endocrine

Causes

Hypothyroidism

Hyperadrenocorticism

Diabetes mellitus

Adrenal sex hormone deficiency (Alopecia X)

Growth hormone deficiency (pituitary dwarfism)

Growth hormone-responsive dermatosis in adult dogs

Castration-responsive dermatosis

Hyperestrogenism

- Sertoli cell tumor (male dog)
- Intact female dog

Hypoestrogenism (poorly understood)

- Estrogen-responsive dermatosis of spayed female dogs
- Feline endocrine alopecia

Hypoandrogenism

- Testosterone-responsive dermatosis (male dog)
- Feline endocrine alopecia

Telogen defluxion (effluvium): often after recent pregnancy or diestrus

Progestin excess (excess of progesterone or 17-hydroxyprogesterone)

Clinical Findings

Nonspecific Features of Endocrine Disease

Bilaterally symmetric alopecia

Follicular dilation, follicular keratosis, follicular atrophy

Orthokeratotic hyperkeratosis

Predominance of telogen hair follicles

Sebaceous gland atrophy

Epidermal atrophy

Thin dermis

Epidermal melanosis

Dermal collagen atrophy

Features Suggestive of Specific Endocrine Disorder
Hypothyroidism
- Vacuolated and/or hypertrophied arrector pili muscles, increased dermal mucin content, thick dermis

Hyperadrenocorticism
- Calcinosis cutis, comedones, absence of erector pili muscles

Hyposomatotropism
- Decreased amount and size of dermal elastin fibers

Growth hormone and castration-responsive dermatoses
- Excessive trichilemmal keratinization (flame follicles)

Claw Disorders

Differential Diagnosis for Abnormal Claws

Bacterial Claw Infection—almost always secondary to an underlying cause
- Trauma—usually one claw affected
- Hypothyroidism
- Hyperadrenocorticism
- Allergies
- Autoimmune disorders
- Symmetrical lupoid onychodystrophy
- Neoplasia

Fungal Claw Infection
- Typically caused by dermatophytes

Symmetrical Lupoid Onychodystrophy
- Suspected to be immune mediated. German shepherds and Rottweilers may be predisposed. Acute onset of claw loss, initially 1-2 but eventually all claws slough. Replacement claws are misshapen, soft or brittle, discolored, and friable and usually slough again. Feet are painful and pruritic. Paronychia is uncommon unless secondary bacterial infection is present.

Drug Eruption

Vasculitis

Diagnostic Tests for Abnormal Claws

- Cytology—suppurative to pyogranulomatous inflammation with bacteria
- Bacterial culture of exudates from claw or claw fold. Mixed infections common. *Staphylococcus* spp. usually isolated
- Fungal culture—*Trichophyton* spp. most commonly isolated but may also see *Microsporum* spp. or *Malassezia* spp.
- Radiography—rule out osteomyelitis

- Dermatohistopathology—(P3 amputation), only recommended to rule out neoplasia. With symmetric lupoid onychodystrophy, see basal cell hydropic degeneration, degeneration or apoptosis of individual keratinocytes in the basal layer, pigmentary incontinence, and lichenoid interface dermatitis. Systemic lupoid onychodystrophy is most commonly diagnosed by typical history and clinical signs along with ruling out other differentials.

Erosions and Ulcerations of Skin or Mucous Membranes

Differential Diagnosis, Dogs

Excoriation from Any Pruritic Skin Disease

Infection

Bacterial Pyoderma
Surface (pyotraumatic moist dermatitis, intertrigo)
Deep (folliculitis, furunculosis, bacterial stomatitis)

Fungal
Yeast infection (*Malassezia pachydermatis, Candida* spp.)
Dermatophytosis
Systemic fungal infection (blastomycosis, coccidioidomycosis, cryptococcosis, histoplasmosis, others)
Subcutaneous mycoses (pythiosis, zygomycosis, phaeohyphomycosis, sporotrichosis, eumycotic mycetoma, others)

Parasitic
Demodicosis

Neoplasia
Squamous cell carcinoma
Epitheliotrophic lymphoma

Metabolic Derangements
Uremia/renal failure
Necrolytic migratory erythema
Calcinosis cutis (hyperadrenocorticism)

Physical/Chemical Injury
Drug reactions
Urine scald
Thermal injury (burn, freeze)
Solar injury

Immune-Mediated Disorders
Discoid lupus erythematosus (DLE)
Pemphigus

Uveodermatologic syndrome

Miscellaneous autoimmune subepidermal vesiculobullous diseases (bullous pemphigoid, epidermolysis acquisita, linear IgA bullous disease, mucocutaneous pemphigoid, bullous systemic lupus type 1)

Miscellaneous

Arthropod bites

Dermatomyositis

Dystrophic epidermolysis bullosa, junctional epidermolysis bullosa

Idiopathic ulceration of Collies

Toxic epidermal necrolysis, erythema multiforme

Differential Diagnosis, Cats

Infection

Viral

Calicivirus

Herpesvirus

Bacterial

Atypical mycobacteriosis

Fungal

Cryptococcosis

Systemic and subcutaneous mycoses

Sporotrichosis

Neoplasia

Squamous cell carcinomas (especially white, outdoor cats)

Fibrosarcoma

Cutaneous lymphoma

Metabolic Derangements

Uremia/renal disease

Physical/Chemical Injury

Thermal

Drug reactions

Immune-Mediated Disorders

Bullous pemphigoid

Pemphigus foliaceus

Plasma cell pododermatitis

Toxic epidermal necrolysis

Inflammatory/Allergic Disorders

Eosinophilic plaque

Indolent ulcer

Arthropod bites

Miscellaneous/Idiopathic
Dystrophic epidermolysis bullosa
Idiopathic ulceration of dorsal neck
Junctional epidermolysis bullosa

Folliculitis

Differential Diagnosis

Superficial Folliculitis
Inflammation of hair follicles
- Bacterial pyoderma
- Fungal (dermatophytosis)
- Parasitic (demodicosis, *Pelodera* dermatitis)

Deep Folliculitis/Furunculosis
Inflammation of hair follicles with subsequent
follicular rupture into dermis and subcutaneous tissues
- Deep pyodermas

Otitis Externa, Chronic

Primary Causes

Allergy
Atopy
Adverse reactions to foods
Contact dermatitis

Parasites
Otodectes cynotis
Notoedres cati
Sarcoptes scabiei
Demodex spp.
Chiggers
Flies
Ticks (spinous ear tick)

Dermatophytes

Endocrine Disorders
Hypothyroidism

Foreign Bodies
Foxtails, hair, etc.

Glandular Conditions
Ceruminous gland hyperplasia
Sebaceous gland hyperplasia or hypoplasia
Altered type or rate of secretions

Autoimmune Diseases
Systemic lupus erythematosus (SLE)
Pemphigus foliaceus/erythematosus
Cold agglutinin disease
Juvenile cellulitis

Viruses
Distemper

Miscellaneous
Solar dermatitis
Frostbite
Vasculitis/vasculopathy
Eosinophilic dermatitis
Sterile eosinophilic folliculitis
Relapsing polychondritis

Predisposing Factors

Conformation
Stenotic canals
Hair in canals
Pendulous pinnae
Hairy, concave pinna

Excessive Moisture
Swimmer's ear
High-humidity climate

Excessive Cerumen Production
Secondary to underlying disease
Primary (idiopathic)

Treatment Effects
Trauma from cotton swabs
Topical irritants
Superinfections from altering microflora

Obstructive Ear Disease
Polyps
Granulomas
Tumors

Systemic Disease
Immunosuppression
Debilitation
Negative catabolic states

Perpetuating Factors

Bacteria (most commonly *Staphylococcus* spp., *Streptococcus* spp., *Pseudomonas* spp., *Proteus*, *Escherichia coli*)

Yeast *(Malassezia pachydermatis)*

Progressive Pathologic Changes
Hyperkeratosis
Hyperplasia
Epithelial folds
Apocrine gland hypertrophy
Hidradenitis
Fibrosis

Otitis Media
Purulent
Caseated or keratinous
Cholesteatoma
Proliferative
Destructive osteomyelitis

Parasitic Dermatoses

Classification

Fleas (*Ctenocephalides felis* most common)
Flea infestation
Flea allergy dermatitis
• Caudal distribution of lesions (dogs)
• Miliary dermatitis (cats)

Demodicosis
Follicular infection *(Demodex canis, Demodex felis)*
Epidermal infection (*Demodex gatoi*, short-tailed demodectic mite of dogs)

Sarcoptic Mange
Sarcoptes scabiei (dogs, rarely cats)
Notoedres cati (cats, rarely dogs)

Ear Mites
Otodectes cynotis (common in both dogs and cats)

Cheyletiellosis
Cheyletiella yasguri (primary host is dogs)
C. blakei (primary host is cats)

C. parasitovorax (primary host is rabbits)
All *Cheyletiella* species freely contagious from one species to another

Chiggers

Larval stage (six-legged bright red or orange) is the parasitic stage; nymph and adult are free living.

Ticks

Brown dog tick *(Rhipicephalus sanguineus)*
American dog tick *(Dermacentor variabilis)*
Rocky Mountain wood tick *(Dermacentor andersoni)*
Lone star tick *(Amblyomma americanum)*
Deer tick *(Ixodes dammini):* primary vector of *Borrelia burgdorferi*
Spinous ear tick *(Otobius megnini)*

Lice

Sucking lice of dogs *(Linognathus setosus)*
Biting lice of dogs *(Trichodectes canis, Heterodoxus springer)*
Lice of cats *(Felicola subrostrata)*

Insects of Order Diptera

Mosquitoes: eosinophilic dermatitis (especially cats)
Black flies, stable flies, horn flies, houseflies: attack ear pinnae of dogs
Myiasis (development of fly larvae in skin or haircoat): screwworm, blow flies, flesh flies
Cuterebra fly larva

Helminth Parasites

Hookworm dermatitis *(Ancylostoma, Uncinaria)*
Pelodera dermatitis *(Pelodera strongyloides)*
Dracunculiasis *(Dracunculus insignis)*

Pigmentation

Differential Diagnosis for Changes in Skin Pigmentation

Hypopigmentation

Vitiligo (Tervuren, Rottweiler, Doberman Pinscher, Newfoundland, Collie, German Shorthaired Pointer, Old English Sheepdog, Siamese cat)
Uveodermatologic syndrome (northern breeds such as Siberian Husky, Samoyed, Akita)
Acquired idiopathic hypopigmentation of nose (Labrador Retriever, Golden Retriever, Malamute, Siberian Husky, Samoyed, Poodle, German Shepherd)

Discoid lupus (German Shepherd, Collie, others)
Dermatomyositis (Collie, Shetland Sheepdog, Beauceron Shepherd)

Hyperpigmentation

Postinflammatory Hyperpigmentation
Any Chronic Pruritic Skin Disease
Atopy
Adverse food reactions
Pyoderma
Malassezia dermatitis
Sarcoptic mange
Erythema multiforme
Many others

Demodicosis

Endocrinopathies
Hypothyroidism
Hyperadrenocortism

Dermatophytosis

Nevus

Lentigo

Neoplasia (melanoma)

Pyoderma

Differential Diagnosis

Surface Pyoderma
Pyotraumatic dermatitis (acute moist dermatitis, "hot spot")
Intertrigo (skin fold dermatitis)

Superficial Pyoderma
Impetigo (subcorneal pustules of sparsely haired skin)
- Puppy pyoderma
Bullous impetigo
- Hyperadrenocorticism, hypothyroidism, diabetes mellitus
Mucocutaneous pyoderma
- Dogs (German Shepherds predisposed)
Superficial bacterial folliculitis
- Staphylococcus pseudintermedius most common
- Local trauma secondary to pruritus (allergy, fleas, scabies, demodicosis, etc.)
Dermatophilosis (rare, actinomycotic superficial crusting dermatitis) methicillin-resistant *Staphylococcus pseudintermedius*

Deep Pyoderma

Always secondary to predisposing problem

Localized lesion (laceration, penetrating wound, animal bite, foreign body)

Generalized (suspect underlying systemic disease)

Clinical syndromes associated with deep pyoderma

- Deep folliculitis, furunculosis, cellulitis
- Pyotraumatic folliculitis
- Muzzle folliculitis and furunculosis
- Pododermatitis (interdigital pyoderma)
- German Shepherd dog folliculitis, furunculosis, cellulitis
- Acral lick furunculosis
- Anaerobic cellulites
- Subcutaneous abscesses
- Bacterial pseudomycetoma
- Mycobacterial granulomas
  - Cutaneous tuberculosis (*Mycobacterium tuberculosis, M. bovis*)
  - Feline leprosy (*M. lepraemurium*)
  - Opportunistic mycobacterial granulomas
- Actinomycosis
- Actinobacillosis
- Nocardiosis

Miscellaneous Bacterial Infections

Brucellosis, plague, borreliosis, *trichomycosis axillaris,* L-form infections

Endocrinologic and Metabolic Disorders

Acromegaly

In dogs, acromegaly is caused by endogenous progesterone from the luteal phase of the estrous cycle or by exogenous progesterone used for estrous prevention. Elevated progesterone, in turn, stimulates excessive growth hormone secretion of mammary origin. In cats, acromegaly is caused by a pituitary adenoma, usually a macroadenoma, which secretes excessive amounts of growth hormone. Physical changes are less pronounced in cats than in dogs.

Clinical Findings, Dogs

Hypertrophy of mouth, tongue, and pharynx
Thick skin folds, myxedema, hypertrichosis
Prognathism
Wide interdental spacing
Visceral organomegaly
Insulin-resistant diabetes mellitus
Polyuria
Polyphagia
Elevated alkaline phosphatase

115

Clinical Findings, Cats

Physical changes most pronounced on head, but all the physical changes listed for dogs may be seen.

Insulin-resistant diabetes mellitus (severe)

Degenerative arthropathy/lameness

Polyuria/polydipsia

Polyphagia

Panting

Lethargy/exercise intolerance

Dyspnea secondary to hypertrophic cardiomyopathy and heart failure

Neurologic signs when macroadenoma becomes large

- Lethargy, stupor
- Adipsia
- Anorexia
- Temperature deregulation
- Circling
- Seizures
- Pituitary dysfunction
  - Hypogonadism
  - Hypothyroidism
  - Hypoadrenocorticism (feline acromegaly may also coexist with pituitary-dependent hyperadrenocorticism)

Adrenal Tumors

Differential Diagnosis

Nonfunctional Adrenal Tumor (dog, rarely cat)

No hormone secreted

Diagnosis by exclusion

Histopathology

Functional Adrenocortical Tumor

Cortisol-Secreting Tumor

Hyperadrenocorticism (Cushing syndrome) (dog, rarely cat)

Diagnosis by adrenocorticotropic hormone (ACTH) stimulation test, low-dose dexamethasone suppression test, adrenal ultrasound, CT scan

Aldosterone-Secreting Tumor

Hyperaldosteronism (Conn syndrome) (cat, rarely dog)

Diagnosis by assessing Na/K, ACTH stimulation test (measure aldosterone)

Progesterone-Secreting Tumor

Mimics hyperadrenocorticism (cat, less commonly dog)

Diagnosis by measuring serum progesterone

Steroid Hormone Precursor–Secreting Tumor

17-hydroxyprogesterone

Mimics hyperadrenocorticism (dog)

Diagnosis by ACTH stimulation test (measure steroid hormone precursors)

Deoxycorticosterone

Mimics hyperadrenocorticism (dog)

Diagnosis by ACTH stimulation test (measure steroid hormone precursors)

Functional Adrenomedullary Tumor

Epinephrine-Secreting Tumor

Pheochromocytosis (dog, rarely cat)

Diagnosis by exclusion, histopathology

Cretinism (Hypothyroidism in Puppies)

Clinical Findings

Dwarfism

Short, broad skull with short thick neck

Enlarged cranium

Shortened limbs

Shortened mandible

Mental dullness

Alopecia

Retention of puppy coat

Kyphosis

Inappetence

Hypothermia

Constipation

Gait abnormalities

Delayed dental eruption

Macroglossia

Dry coat

Thick skin

Lethargy

Dyspnea

Goiter

Diabetes Insipidus

Differential Diagnosis

Features of diabetes insipidus include polyuria, polydipsia, and a near-continuous demand for water. Only the following three disorders can cause the degree of polyuria and dilute urine seen with diabetes insipidus:

- Central diabetes insipidus
- Nephrogenic diabetes insipidus
- Primary polydipsia

Causes in Dogs and Cats

Central Diabetes Insipidus

Idiopathic

Traumatic

Neoplasia

- Primary pituitary neoplasm
- Meningioma
- Craniopharyngioma
- Chromophobe adenoma
- Chromophobe adenocarcinoma
- Metastatic neoplasia

Pituitary malformation

Cysts

Inflammation

Parasitic lesions

Complication of pituitary surgery

Familial?

Nephrogenic Diabetes Insipidus

Polyuria caused by nonresponsiveness to antidiuretic hormone (ADH).

Primary idiopathic

Primary familial (Husky)

Secondary acquired

- Renal insufficiency or failure
- Hyperadrenocorticism
- Hypoadrenocorticism
- Hepatic insufficiency
- Pyometra
- Hypercalcemia
- Hypokalemia
- Postobstructive diuresis
- Diabetes mellitus
- Normoglycemic glucosuria
- Hyperthyroidism
- Iatrogenic or drug induced
- Renal medullary solute washout

Diabetic Ketoacidosis

Clinical Findings

No signs may be seen early with diabetic ketoacidosis.

Historical Findings
   Lethargy
   Anorexia
   Vomiting

Physical Examination Findings
   Dehydration
   Depression
   Weakness
   Tachypnea
   Vomiting
   Acetone odor on breath
   Slow, deep breaths (secondary to metabolic acidosis)
   Abdominal pain/abdominal distension secondary to
      concurrent pancreatitis

Clinicopathologic Findings
   Hyperglycemia
   Metabolic acidosis
   Hypercholesterolemia/lipemia
   Increased alkaline phosphatase (ALP)
   Increased alanine aminotransferase (ALT)
   Increased blood urea nitrogen (BUN)/creatinine
   Hyponatremia
   Hypochloremia
   Hypokalemia
   Increased amylase/lipase
   Hyperosmolality
   Glycosuria
   Ketonuria
   Urinary tract infection

Diabetes Mellitus

Potential Factors in Etiopathogenesis

   Obesity
   Pancreatitis
   Immune-mediated insulitis
   Concurrent hormonal disease
   • Hyperadrenocorticism
   • Diestrus-induced excess of growth hormone
   • Hypothyroidism
   Genetics (dog, possibly cat)
   Drugs
   • Glucocorticoids
   • Megestrol acetate (cat)
   Infection

Concurrent illness
- Renal insufficiency
- Cardiac disease

Hyperlipidemia (dog, possibly cat)

Islet amyloidosis

Clinicopathologic Abnormalities, Uncomplicated Diabetes Mellitus

Complete Blood Count
Often normal

Leukocytosis if pancreatitis or infection present

Serum Chemistry
Hyperglycemia

Mild increase in alkaline phosphatase (ALP) and alanine aminotransferase (ALT)

Hypercholesterolemia/hypertriglyceridemia

Urinalysis
Urine specific gravity normal to mildly decreased (>1.025)

Glycosuria

Variable ketonuria

Bacteriuria

Proteinuria

Ancillary Tests
Increased amylase/lipase if pancreatitis present

Normal serum trypsin-like immunoreactivity (TLI)

Low TLI with exocrine pancreatic insufficiency

High TLI with acute pancreatitis

Normal to high TLI with chronic pancreatitis

Low to normal serum insulin with insulin-dependent diabetes mellitus

Low, normal, or increased serum insulin with non–insulin-dependent diabetes mellitus

Potential Complications

Common
Iatrogenic hypoglycemia

Polyuria/polydipsia

Weight loss

Cataracts (dog)

Anterior uveitis

Bacterial infections (especially urinary tract infection)

Ketoacidosis

Pancreatitis

Peripheral neuropathy (cat)

Hepatic lipidosis

Uncommon
Peripheral neuropathy (dog)
Glomerulopathy
Glomerulosclerosis
Retinopathy
Exocrine pancreatic insufficiency
Gastric paresis
Diabetic diarrhea
Diabetic dermatopathy

Causes of Insulin Resistance or Ineffectiveness in Dogs and Cats

Caused by Insulin Therapy
Improper administration
Inadequate dose
Inactive insulin
Diluted insulin
Somogyi effect
Inappropriate insulin administration
Impaired insulin absorption
Antiinsulin antibody excess

Caused by Concurrent Disorder
Obesity
Diabetogenic drugs
Hyperadrenocorticism
Hypothyroidism (dog)
Hyperthyroidism (cat)
Urinary tract infection
Oral infections
Chronic inflammation/pancreatitis
Diestrus (bitch)
Acromegaly (cat)
Renal insufficiency
Hepatic insufficiency
Cardiac insufficiency
Glucagonoma
Pheochromocytoma
Exocrine pancreatic insufficiency
Hyperlipidemia
Neoplasia

Clinical Findings Associated with Insulin-Secreting Tumors

Seizures
Weakness
Collapse
Ataxia

Polyphagia
Weight gain
Muscle fasciculations
Posterior weakness (neuropathy)
Lethargy
Nervousness
Unusual behavior

Gastrinoma (Zollinger-Ellison Syndrome)

Clinical Findings

Clinical Signs
Vomiting
Weight loss
Anorexia
Diarrhea
Gastric and duodenal ulceration
Hematochezia
Hematemesis
Melena
Obstipation
Lethargy/depression
Abdominal pain
Esophageal pain and ulceration
Regurgitation
Fever
Polydipsia
Thin body condition
Pallor

Clinicopathologic Findings
Regenerative anemia
Hypoproteinemia
Neutrophilic leukocytosis
Hypoalbuminemia
Hypocalcemia
Mild increases in hepatic enzymes
Hypochloremia
Hypokalemia
Hyponatremia
Metabolic acidosis
Metabolic acidosis (secondary to vomiting)
Hyperglycemia, hypoglycemia (uncommon)

Glucagonoma

Clinical Findings in Dogs

Clinical Signs

Necrolytic migratory erythema (crusting skin rash of elbows, hocks, nose, scrotum, flank, ventral abdomen, distal extremities, and mucocutaneous junctions of mouth, eyes, prepuce and vulva)

Footpad lesions

Glucose intolerance/diabetes mellitus (caused by excess glycogenolysis and gluconeogenesis)

Oral ulcerations

Lethargy

Weight loss

Decreased appetite

Muscle atrophy

Peripheral lymphadenopathy

Clinicopathologic Findings

Hyperglycemia

Nonregenerative anemia

Increased hepatic enzymes

Decreased albumin

Decreased globulin

Decreased blood urea nitrogen (BUN)

Decreased cholesterol

Glucosuria

Abdominal ultrasound lesions

- Increased echogenicity of portal and hepatic vein walls
- Diffuse hyperechogenicity
- Multiple small hypoechoic foci

Hyperadrenocorticism

Clinical Findings

Potential Clinical Signs

Polyuria/polydipsia

Alopecia

Pendulous abdomen

Hepatomegaly

Polyphagia

Muscle weakness

Muscle atrophy

Pyoderma

Comedones
Panting
Pacing/restlessness
Hyperpigmentation
Systemic hypertension
Testicular atrophy
Anestrus
Calcinosis cutis
Facial nerve paralysis
Pulmonary thromboembolism

Potential Clinicopathologic Findings

Urinary tract infection/pyelonephritis
Decreased urine specific gravity
Increased serum alkaline phosphatase (ALP)
Increased alanine aminotransferase (ALT)
Hypercholesterolemia
Hypertriglyceridemia
Hyperglycemia (mild to moderate)
Diabetes mellitus (uncommon)
Increased serum bile acids
Decreased BUN and creatinine (secondary to diuresis)
Hypophosphatemia
Stress leukogram
- Neutrophilia
- Lymphopenia
- Eosinopenia
- Monocytosis
Thrombocytosis
Mild erythrocytosis
Decreased total serum thyroxine (T_4) or free T_4
Urolithiasis

Hyperglycemia

Differential Diagnosis

Diabetes mellitus
Stress (physiologic in cat)
Hyperadrenocorticism
Drug therapy
- Glucocorticoids
- Progestagens
- Megestrol acetate
- Thiazide diuretics
Dextrose-containing fluids
Parenteral nutrition

Postprandial effect (diets containing monosaccharides, disaccharides, propylene glycol)
Exocrine pancreatic neoplasia
Pancreatitis
Renal insufficiency
Acromegaly (cat)
Pheochromocytoma (dog)
Diestrus (bitch)
Head trauma

Hypoadrenocorticism

Potential Clinical Findings

Clinical Signs
Lethargy/depression
Episodic weakness
Vomiting
Anorexia
Waxing and waning illness
Weight loss/failure to gain weight
Bradycardia
Dehydration/hypovolemia
Diarrhea
Polyuria or polydipsia
Collapse
Syncope
Restlessness/shaking/shivering
Regurgitation
Muscle cramping
Gastrointestinal hemorrhage/melena
Abdominal pain

Potential Clinicopathologic Findings
Hyponatremia
Hyperkalemia
Hypochloremia
Decreased sodium/potassium ratio (<24:1)
Azotemia
- Increased blood urea nitrogen (BUN)
- Increased creatinine
- Increased phosphate
Decreased bicarbonate and total CO_2 concentrations
Hypercalcemia
Hypoglycemia
Hypoalbuminemia
Increased hepatic enzymes

Metabolic acidosis
Lymphocytosis
Eosinophilia
Relative neutropenia
Anemia (usually nonregenerative)
Variable urine specific gravity (<1.030)

Hypoglycemia

Differential Diagnosis

Excess Secretion of Insulin or Insulin-Like Factors
Insulinoma
Extrapancreatic tumor
Islet cell hyperplasia

Decreased Glucose Production
Toy breeds
Neonates
Malnutrition
Pregnancy
Fasting
Hypoadrenocorticism
Hypopituitarism
Growth hormone deficiency
Liver disease (portal caval shunt, chronic fibrosis/cirrhosis)
Glycogen storage diseases

Excess Glucose Consumption
Sepsis
Extreme exercise

Drug-Associated Causes
Insulin
Oral hypoglycemics
Many other drugs reported to cause hypoglycemia in humans

Spurious
Blood cells not promptly separated from serum

Hyponatremia/Hyperkalemia

Differential Diagnosis

Hypoadrenocorticism

Renal or Urinary Tract Disease
Urethral obstruction
Acute renal failure
Chronic oliguric or anuric renal failure

Postobstructive diuresis
Nephrotic syndrome

Severe Gastrointestinal Disease

Parasitic infestation
- Whipworm (trichuriasis)
- Roundworm (ascariasis)
- Hookworm (ancylostomiasis)

Salmonellosis
Viral enteritis
- Parvovirus
- Canine distemper virus

Gastric dilatation/volvulus
Gastrointestinal perforation
Severe malabsorption
Hemorrhagic gastroenteritis
Pancreatic disease

Severe Hepatic Failure

Cirrhosis
Neoplasia

Severe Metabolic or Respiratory Acidosis

Congestive Heart Failure

Massive Release of Potassium into Extracellular Fluid

Crush injury
Aortic thrombosis
Rhabdomyolysis
- Heat stroke
- Exertional

Massive sepsis
Massive hemolysis

Pleural Effusion

Pregnancy

Lymphangiosarcoma

Pseudohyperkalemia

Akitas and related breeds
Severe leukocytosis (>100,000/mm^3)
Severe thrombocytosis (>1 million/mm^3)

Diabetes Mellitus

Primary Polydipsia

Inappropriate Antidiuretic Hormone (ADH) Secretion

Drug Induced

Potassium-sparing diuretics
Nonsteroidal antiinflammatory drugs (NSAIDs)

Angiotensin-converting enzyme (ACE) inhibitors
Potassium-containing fluids

Insulinoma

Differential Diagnosis for Insulin-Secreting Beta-Cell Neoplasia

Excess Insulin or Insulin-Like Factors
Insulinoma
Extrapancreatic tumor
Islet cell hyperplasia

Decreased Glucose Production
Hypoadrenocorticism
Hypopituitarism
Growth hormone deficiency
Liver disease
Glycogen storage diseases
Neonates
Toy breeds
Fasting
Malnutrition
Pregnancy

Excess Glucose Consumption
Sepsis
Extreme exercise

Drug-Associated Causes
Insulin
Oral hypoglycemics (sulfonylurea)
Salicylates (e.g., aspirin)
Acetaminophen
β-blockers
$β_2$-agonists
Ethanol
Monoamine oxidase inhibitors
Tricyclic antidepressants
Angiotensin-converting enzyme (ACE) inhibitors
Antibiotics (e.g., tetracycline)
Lidocaine overdose
Lithium

Factitious Hypoglycemia
Failure to separate blood cells from serum promptly
Severe polycythemia or leukocytosis when serum separation delayed

Parathyroidism

Hyperparathyroidism, Primary—Clinical Findings

Clinical Signs
Polyuria/polydipsia
Weight loss
Anorexia
Lethargy, listlessness
Urinary tract infection (UTI)
Urolithiasis
Vomiting
Constipation
Mental dullness, obtundation, coma
Weakness, muscle wasting, shivering

Clinicopathologic Findings
Hypercalcemia
Increased ionized calcemia
Low normal to low serum phosphorus
Decreased urine specific gravity
Hematuria
Pyuria
Crystalluria
Bacteriuria

Hypoparathyroidism—Clinical Findings

Clinical Signs
Seizures
Facial rubbing, biting at feet
Splinted abdomen
Stiff gait
Intermittent lameness
Muscle fasciculations, cramping, tremors
Fever
Paroxysmal tachyarrhythmias
Muffled heart sounds
Weak pulses
Disorientation

Clinicopathologic Findings
Hypocalcemia
Hyperphosphatemia
Decreased serum parathyroid hormone concentration

Electrocardiographic Findings
Deep, wide T waves
Prolonged QT interval
Bradycardia

Pheochromocytoma

Clinical Findings

Intermittent weakness
Intermittent collapse
Panting
Tachypnea
Seizures
Tachycardia
Lethargy
Inappetence
Cardiac arrhythmias
Restlessness
Exercise intolerance
Weak pulses
Vomiting
Diarrhea
Weight loss
Muscle wasting
Polyuria/polydipsia
Abdominal distension
Rear limb edema
Pale mucous membranes
Abdominal pain
Hemorrhage (epistaxis, surgical incision sites)
Palpable abdominal mass

Pituitary Dwarfism

Clinical Findings

Musculoskeletal Signs
Stunted growth
Delayed growth plate closure
Thin skeleton
Immature facial features
Square, chunky contour as adult
Bone deformities
Delayed dental eruption

Dermatologic Signs
Soft, woolly haircoat
Lack of guard hairs
Alopecia; bilaterally symmetric trunk, neck, and proximal
  extremities
Hyperpigmentation
Thin, fragile skin

Wrinkles
Scales
Comedones
Papules
Pyoderma
Seborrhea sicca
Retention of secondary hairs

Reproductive Signs
Testicular atrophy
Unilateral or bilateral cryptorchidism
Flaccid penile sheath
Failure to have estrous cycles

Other Signs
Mental dullness
Shrill, puppy-like bark
Signs of secondary hypothyroidism
Signs of secondary adrenal insufficiency

Thyroid Disease

Hyperthyroidism, Feline—Clinical Findings

Clinical Signs
Weight loss/thin body condition
Polyphagia
Hyperactivity
Palpable thyroid nodule (goiter)
Tachycardia
Vomiting
Cardiac murmur
Premature beats
Gallop rhythm
Aggressiveness
Panting
Pacing
Restlessness
Increased nail growth
Alopecia
Polyuria/polydipsia
Diarrhea
Increased fecal volume
Muscle weakness
Congestive heart failure (CHF)
Dyspnea
Ventroflexion of neck

Unkempt coat/alopecia
Tremor
Weakness
Anorexia

Hypothyroidism, Canine—Clinical Findings

Clinical Signs

Lethargy/exercise intolerance
Weight gain
Cold intolerance
Mental dullness
Dermatologic signs

- Alopecia
- Superficial pyoderma
- Seborrhea sicca or oleosa
- Dry, scaly skin
- Changes in haircoat quality and color
- Hyperkeratosis
- Hyperpigmentation
- Comedones
- Hypertrichosis
- Ceruminous otitis
- Myxedema (cutaneous mucinosis)
- Poor wound healing
- Slow regrowth of hair

Reproductive abnormalities

- Male: decreased libido, testicular atrophy, hypospermia
- Female: delayed estrus, silent estrus, failure to cycle, abortion, small litters, uterine inertia, weak or stillborn puppies

Peripheral neuropathies

- Generalized peripheral neuropathies
- Specific peripheral neuropathies (especially cranial nerves, facial, trigeminal, vestibulocochlear)

Cerebral dysfunction (myxedema coma [rare])
Cardiovascular signs

- Sinus bradycardia, weak apex beat, low QRS voltages, inverted T waves, hypercholesterolemia leading to atherosclerosis (rare)

Ocular abnormalities (corneal lipidosis, corneal ulceration, uveitis, secondary glaucoma, lipemia retinalis, retinal detachment, and keratoconjunctivitis sicca reported, but causal relationship not proven)

Clinicopathologic Changes
Nonregenerative anemia
Hypercholesterolemia
Hypertriglyceridemia
Mild increases in hepatic enzymes

Gastroenterologic Disorders

Chronic Constipation, Feline

Differential Diagnosis

Neuromuscular Dysfunction
- Colonic smooth muscle: idiopathic megacolon, aging
- Spinal cord disease: lumbosacral disease, cauda equina syndrome, sacral spinal cord deformities (Manx cat)
- Hypogastric or pelvic nerve disorders: traumatic injury, malignancy, dysautonomia

Mechanical Obstruction
- Intraluminal: foreign material, neoplasia, rectal diverticula, perineal hernia, anorectal strictures
- Intramural: neoplasia
- Extraluminal: pelvic fractures, neoplasia

Inflammation
- Perianal fistula, proctitis, anal sac abscess, anorectal foreign bodies, perianal bite wounds

Metabolic and Endocrine
- Metabolic: dehydration, hypokalemia, hypercalcemia
- Endocrine: hypothyroidism, obesity, nutritional secondary hyperparathyroidism

Environmental and Behavioral
- Soiled litter box, inactivity, hospitalization, change in environment

Diarrhea

Causes of Diarrhea

Gastrointestinal Disease
- Diffuse gastrointestinal disease (e.g., inflammation or lymphoma)
- Gastric disease (achlorhydria, dumping syndromes)
- Intestinal disease (primary small intestinal disease, primary large intestinal disease, dietary-induced such as food poisoning, gluttony, or sudden change of diet)

Nongastrointestinal Disease
- Pancreatic disease (exocrine pancreatic insufficiency, pancreatitis, pancreatic carcinoma, gastrinoma or Zollinger-Ellison syndrome)
- Liver disease (hepatocellular failure, intrahepatic and extrahepatic cholestasis)
- Endocrine disease (classical hypoadrenocorticism, atypical hypoadrenocorticism, hyperthyroidism, hypothyroidism)
- Renal disease (uremia, nephrotic syndrome)
- Polysystemic infection (e.g., distemper, leptospirosis, infectious canine hepatitis in dogs, FIP, FeLV, FIV in cats)
- Miscellaneous (toxemias such as pyometra and peritonitis, congestive heart failure, autoimmune disease, metastatic neoplasia, various toxins and drugs)

Classification of Diarrhea

Mechanistic
- Secretory
- Osmotic
- Permeability (exudative)
- Dysmotility
- Mixed

Temporal
- Acute
- Chronic

Anatomic
- Extraintestinal
- Small intestinal
- Large intestinal
- Diffuse

Pathophysiologic
- Biochemical
- Allergic
- Inflammatory
- Neoplastic

Etiologic
- Bacteria
- Dietary
- Fungal
- Idiopathic
- Parasitic
- Viral

Causal
- Exocrine pancreatic insufficiency, salmonellosis, lymphoma, other

Clinical
- Acute, nonfatal, mild, self-limiting
- Acute, severe potentially fatal
- Acute systemic disease
- Chronic
- Chronic protein-losing

Dental and Oral Cavity Diseases

Differential Diagnosis

Trauma
Fractures
- Crown
- Root
- Mandible
- Maxillary

Avulsion
Pulp injury
Temporomandibular luxation

Caries

Feline Dental Resorptive Lesions

Periodontal Disease
Gingivitis
Gingival recession
Bone loss, osteomyelitis
Tooth loss

Tooth Root Abscess

Oronasal Fistula

Stomatitis (Faucitis, Glossitis, Pharyngitis)

Feline immunodeficiency virus, feline leukemia virus, feline syncytium-forming virus

Feline calicivirus, feline herpesvirus, feline infectious peritonitis

Candidiasis

Uremia

Trauma (foreign objects, caustic agents, electric cord bite)

Autoimmune disease (pemphigus, lupus, idiopathic vasculitis, toxic epidermal necrolysis)

Feline idiopathic gingivitis/pharyngitis

Neoplasia

Malignant

Fibrosarcoma

Squamous cell carcinoma

Melanoma

Salivary gland neoplasms

Benign

Epulis

- Fibromatous
- Acanthomatous
- Ossifying
- Papilloma
- Fibroma
- Lipoma
- Chondroma
- Osteoma
- Hemangioma
- Hemangiopericytoma
- Histiocytoma

Eosinophilic Granuloma Complex

Linear granuloma

Eosinophilic ulcer (usually on maxillary lips)

Sialocele

Diseases of the Tongue

Differential Diagnosis

Trauma

- Mechanical injury (sharp objects)
- Chemical injury
- Electric shock (electric cord)

- Foreign body (plant material, porcupine quill, linear foreign bodies)
- Sublingual hyperplastic tissue (gum chewer's disease)

Viral
- Calicivirus
- Herpes virus
- Papillomavirus

Neoplasia
- Malignant melanoma
- Squamous cell carcinoma
- Benign tumors (lipoma, plasma cell tumor, granular cell tumors, fibroma)

Metabolic Disease (Uremia)

Sublingual Mucocele (Ranula)

Immune Mediated
- Mucous membrane pemphigoid
- Pemphigus vulgaris
- Bullous pemphigoid
- Systemic lupus erythematosus
- Autoimmune vasculopathies (idiopathic, infectious, food allergies, drug reaction, neoplasia)

Eosinophilic granulomas

Contact Mucosal Ulceration from Calculus Contact

Calcinosis Circumscripta

Salivary Gland Disease

Differential Diagnosis

Salivary Neoplasia (more common in cats than dogs)
Adenocarcinoma
Squamous cell carcinoma
Undifferentiated sarcoma
Mucoepidermoid tumor
Malignant mixed tumor
Sarcoma
Acinic cell carcinoma
Adenoid cystic carcinoma

Salivary Mucocele
Sublingual gland most commonly

Sialoadenitis

Sialadenosis

Esophageal Disease

Differential Diagnosis

Congenital

Obstruction

Persistent right aortic arch
Persistent right or left subclavian artery
Other vascular ring anomaly

Idiopathic

Acquired

Obstruction

Foreign body
Cicatrix/stricture
Neoplasia
- Carcinoma
- *Spirocerca lupi*–induced sarcoma
- Leiomyoma of lower esophageal sphincter
- Extraesophageal neoplasia
  - Thyroid carcinoma
  - Pulmonary carcinoma
  - Mediastinal lymphosarcoma

Achalasia of lower esophageal sphincter (rare)
Gastroesophageal intussusception (rare)

Weakness

Myasthenia (generalized or localized)
Hypoadrenocorticism
Esophagitis
Persistent vomiting
Hiatal hernia
Gastroesophageal reflux/anesthesia-associated reflux
Caustic ingestion (doxycycline, disinfectants, chemicals, etc.)
Foreign body
Excess gastric acidity (gastrinoma, mast cell tumor)
Fungal organisms (e.g., pythiosis)

Spirocerca lupi Infection

Myopathies/Neuropathies

Hypothyroidism
Systemic lupus erythematosus (SLE)
Others

Miscellaneous Causes

Lead poisoning
Chagas disease

Canine distemper
Dermatomyositis (principally in Collies)
Dysautonomia
Tetanus

Idiopathic

Stomach Disorders

Differential Diagnosis

Gastritis

Acute Gastritis

Dietary indiscretion
Dietary intolerance or allergy
Foreign body
Drugs and toxins (nonsteroidal antiinflammatory
drugs [NSAIDs], corticosteroids, antibiotics, plants,
cleaners, bleach, heavy metals)
Systemic disease (uremia, hepatic disease,
hypoadrenocorticism)
Parasites (*Ollulanus* spp., *Physaloptera* spp.)
Bacterial (bacterial toxins, *Helicobacter* spp.)

Hemorrhagic Gastroenteritis

Chronic Gastritis

Lymphocytic/plasmacytic gastritis (inflammatory
reaction to a variety of antigens such as *Helicobacter*
spp. or *Physaloptera rara*)
Eosinophilic gastritis (allergic reactions to food
antigens)
Granulomatous gastritis (e.g., *Ollulanus tricuspis*)
Atrophic gastritis

Gastric Outflow Obstruction/Gastric Stasis

Benign muscular pyloric hypertrophy (pyloric stenosis)
Gastric antral mucosal hypertrophy
Foreign body
Idiopathic gastric hypomotility
Bilious vomiting syndrome

Gastric Ulceration/Erosion

Iatrogenic

NSAIDs
Corticosteroids
NSAID/corticosteroid combinations

Foreign Body

Helicobacter **spp.**

Stress Ulceration
    Hypovolemic shock
    Septic shock
    After gastric dilatation/volvulus
    • Neurogenic shock
    Hyperacidity
    • Mast cell tumor
    • Gastrinoma (rare)
    Other causes
    • Hepatic disease
    • Renal disease
    • Hypoadrenocorticism
    • Inflammatory disease

Infiltrative Disease
    Neoplasia
    Inflammatory bowel disease
    Pythiosis (young dogs, southeastern United States)

Gastric Dilatation/Volvulus

Causes of Acute Abdomen

Gastrointestinal (GI) Causes
    Acute pancreatitis
    Gastroenteritis (parvoviral, bacterial, toxic, hemorrhagic gastroenteritis, etc.)
    Gastric dilatation/volvulus
    Intestinal obstruction/intussusception/volvulus
    Colitis
    Obstipation
    Necrosis, rupture, ulceration, or perforation of GI tract
    Surgical wound dehiscence
    Mesenteric torsion
    Duodenocolic ligament entrapment
    Pancreatic abscess
    Pancreatic neoplasia

Hepatobiliary Causes
    Acute hepatitis/cholangiohepatitis
    Biliary obstruction
    Necrotizing cholecystitis
    Hepatic abscess
    Bile peritonitis

Liver lobe torsion
Hepatic trauma/rupture
Hepatobiliary neoplasia

Urogenital Causes

Urethral or ureteral obstruction/rupture
Pyelonephritis
Renal neoplasia
Acute nephrosis/nephritis
Cystic, renal, ureteral, or urethral calculi
Prostatitis/prostatic abscess/prostatic cyst/prostatic
  neoplasia
Dystocia
Pyometra/uterine rupture
Acute metritis
Renal abscess
Testicular torsion
Ovarian cyst, ovarian neoplasia
Uterine torsion
Uroabdomen
Vaginal rupture

Other Causes

Penetrating wound, crush injury
Peritonitis (septic, chemical, urine, bile)
Mesenteric traction (large masses)/lymphadenitis/lymph-
  adenopathy/volvulus/avulsion/artery thrombosis
Hemoabdomen (parenchymatous organ rupture)
Neoplasia
Splenic torsion/abscess/mass/rupture
Strangulated hernia
Adhesions with organ entrapment
Pansteatitis
Retroperitoneal hemorrhage
Evisceration
Surgical contamination

Small Intestinal Disease

Clinical Findings

Diarrhea
Vomiting
Inappetence/anorexia
Malabsorption
Protein-losing enteropathy
Weight loss
Dehydration

Hematemesis
Melena
Polyphagia
Coprophagia
Abdominal distension
Abdominal pain
Borborygmus/flatulence
Ascites
Edema
Shock
Halitosis
Polydipsia
Ileus

Differential Diagnosis

Acute Diarrhea

Acute enteritis
Dietary indiscretion
Enterotoxemia

Infectious Diarrhea

Canine parvoviral enteritis
Clostridial disease
Feline parvoviral enteritis (panleukopenia)
Canine coronaviral enteritis
Feline coronaviral enteritis
Feline leukemia virus–associated panleukopenia
Feline immunodeficiency virus–associated diarrhea
Salmon poisoning *(Neorickettsia helminthoeca)*
Campylobacteriosis
Salmonellosis
Histoplasmosis
Miscellaneous *bacteria (Yersinia enterocolitica, Aeromonas hydrophila, Plesiomonas shigelloides)*
Prototothecosis (algae)

Alimentary Tract Parasites

Roundworms *(Toxocara* spp.)
Hookworms *(Ancylostoma, Uncinaria* spp.)
Tapeworms *(Dipylidium caninum, Taenia* spp., *Mesocestoides* spp.)
Strongyloides stercoralis (in puppies)
Coccidiosis
Cryptosporidia
Giardiasis
Trichomoniasis
Heterobilharzia

Maldigestive Disease
Exocrine pancreatic insufficiency

Malabsorptive Disease
Dietary-responsive disease (allergy, intolerance)
Inflammatory bowel disease (lymphocytic/plasmacytic enteritis canine eosinophilic gastroenteritis)
Feline eosinophilic enteritis/hypereosinophilic syndrome
Granulomatous enteritis
Immunoproliferative enteropathy in Basenjis
Enteropathy in Shar-Peis
Antibiotic-responsive enteropathy

Protein-Losing Enteropathy
Intestinal lymphangiectasia
Protein-losing enteropathy in Soft-Coated Wheaten Terriers

Irritable Bowel Syndrome

Intestinal Obstruction
Simple intestinal obstruction
Incarcerated intestinal obstruction
Mesenteric torsion/volvulus
Linear foreign object

Intussusception
Ileocolic
Jejunojejunal

Short-Bowel Syndrome

Neoplasia
Alimentary lymphoma
Intestinal adenocarcinoma
Intestinal leiomyoma/leiomyosarcoma

Breed Susceptibilities, Dogs

Basenji: lymphocytic/plasmacytic enteritis (immunoproliferative disease)
Beagle: cobalamin deficiency
Border Collie: cobalamin deficiency
German Shepherd: idiopathic antibiotic-responsive small intestinal disease, inflammatory bowel disease (lymphoplasmacytic, eosinophilic)
Giant Schnauzer: defective cobalamin absorption
Irish Setter: gluten-sensitive enteropathy

Lundehund: lymphangiectasia
Retrievers: dietary allergy
Rottweiler: increased susceptibility to parvoviral enteritis
Soft-Coated Wheaten Terrier: protein-losing enteropathy/
  nephropathy
Shar-Pei: lymphocytic/plasmacytic enteritis, cobalamin
  deficiency
Yorkshire Terrier: lymphangiectasia
Toy breeds: hemorrhagic gastroenteritis

Large Intestinal Disease

Differential Diagnosis

Inflammation of Large Intestine
Acute colitis/proctitis
Chronic colitis
- Lymphocytic/plasmacytic colitis
- Eosinophilic enterocolitis
- Chronic ulcerative colitis
- Histiocytic ulcerative colitis (Boxers)
Irritable bowel syndrome

Dietary Intolerance or Food Allergy

Parasites
Whipworms (*Trichuris* spp.)
Tritrichomonas spp. (cats)
Giardiasis
Hookworms (*Ancylostoma* spp.)
Heterobilharzia americanum

Bacterial Colitis
Clostridial colitis
Campylobacter colitis
Escherichia coli
Salmonell a spp.
Brachispira pilosicoli

Fungal Colitis
Histoplasmosis
Pythiosis

Viral Colitis
Feline leukemia virus (FeLV)
Infections secondary to FeLV and feline immunodeficiency
  virus (FIV)

Algae (*Prototheca* spp.)

Cecocolic Intussusception

Rectal Prolapse

Neoplasms of Large Intestine
Adenocarcinoma
Lymphoma
Rectal polyps

Constipation
Pelvic canal obstruction caused by malaligned healing of
pelvic fractures
Benign rectal stricture
Dietary indiscretion leading to constipation
Idiopathic megacolon

Ileus

Causes

Physical
Intestinal obstruction (foreign body, intussusception,
neoplasia, granuloma, torsion, volvulus, incarceration
in hernia)
Overdistension by aerophagia

Metabolic
Uremia
Diabetes mellitus
Hypokalemia
Endotoxemia

Inflammatory
Parvovirus
Peritonitis
Other inflammatory causes

Functional
Abdominal surgery
Peritonitis
Pancreatitis
Ischemia

Neuromuscular
Anticholinergic drugs
Spinal cord injury
Visceral myopathies/neuropathy
Dysautonomia

Malabsorptive Diseases

Causes

Food intolerance or allergy
Parasitism
- Giardiasis

Bacterial overgrowth
Inflammatory bowel disease
- Lymphocytic/plasmacytic enteritis
- Eosinophilic enteritis
- Idiopathic villous atrophy
- Purulent enteritis

Gastrointestinal lymphoma
Lymphangiectasia
Obstruction caused by neoplasia, infection, or inflammation
Portal hypertension
Pythiosis
Exocrine pancreatic insufficiency
Cholestatic liver disease/biliary obstruction
Brush border enzyme deficiencies
Brush border transport protein deficiencies
Hyperthyroidism
Gastric hypersecretion

Perianal Disease

Differential Diagnosis

Perineal hernia
Perianal fistulae
Anal sacculitis
Anal sac impaction
Abscessed anal sac
Anal sac (apocrine gland) adenocarcinoma
Perianal gland tumors
- Adenoma (common)
- Adenosarcoma (rare)

Protein-Losing Enteropathy

Differential Diagnosis

Gastrointestinal Hemorrhage
Hemorrhagic gastroenteritis
Ulceration
Neoplasia

Endoparasites
Giardia spp.
Ancylostoma spp.
Coccidia
Others

Inflammation
Lymphocytic/plasmacytic
Eosinophilic
Granulomatous

Infection
Parvovirus
Salmonellosis
Histoplasmosis
Phycomycosis

Structural
Intussusception

Neoplasia
Lymphosarcoma

Lymphangiectasia
Primary lymphatic disorder
Venous hypertension (e.g., right heart failure)
Hepatic cirrhosis

Fecal Incontinence

Causes

Nonneurologic Disease
Colorectal Disease
Inflammatory bowel disease
Neoplasia
Constipation

Anorectal Disease
Perianal fistula
Neoplasia
Surgery (anal sacculectomy, perianal herniorrhaphy, rectal resection and anastomosis)

Miscellaneous
Decreased mentation
Old age
Severe diarrhea
Irritable bowel disease

Neurologic Disease

Sacral Spinal Cord Disease
Discospondylitis
Neoplasia
Degenerative myelopathy
Congenital vertebral malformation
Sacrococcygeal hypoplasia of Manx cats
Sacral fracture
Sacrococcygeal subluxation
Lumbosacral instability
Lumbrosacral nerve root compression
Meningomyelocele
Viral meningomyelitis
Cauda equina syndrome
Vertebral fracture

Peripheral Neuropathy
Trauma
Penetrating wounds
Repair of perineal hernia
Perineal urethrostomy
Hypothyroidism?
Diabetes mellitus?
Dysautonomia

Central Nervous System
Infectious (distemper, feline infectious peritonitis)
Neoplasia
Vascular compromise

Hematologic Disorders

Anemia

Hemolytic Anemia

Causes/Triggers of Immune-Mediated Hemolytic Anemia

Infection

Viral

Feline leukemia virus (FeLV), feline immunodeficiency virus (FIV), feline peritonitis virus (FIP), chronic upper respiratory or gastrointestinal (GI) disease

Bacterial

Leptospirosis, *Mycoplasma haemophilus* infection, salmonellosis, acute and chronic infections (e.g., abscess, pyometra, discospondylitis)

Parasitic

Babesiosis, anaplasmosis, leishmaniasis, dirofilariasis, ehrlichiosis, *Ancylostoma caninum, Trichuris vulpis* infection, bartonellosis

Immune Disorders

Systemic lupus erythematosus (SLE)
Hypothyroidism
Primary and secondary immunodeficiencies

Drugs/Toxins

Vaccines
Sulfonamides
Methimazole
Procainamide
Cephalosporins
Penicillins
Propylthiouracil
Carprofen
Levamisole

Griseofulvin
Bee-sting envenomation

Oxidants
Acetaminophen
Phenothiazines
Vitamin K
Methylene blue
Methionine
Propylene glycol

Inflammation
Pancreatitis
Prostatitis/cystitis

Neoplasia
Leukemias
Lymphoma
Multiple myeloma
Mast cell tumor
Splenic hemangioma
Solid tumors

Genetic Predisposition
American Cocker Spaniel (most common breed),
English Springer Spaniel, Old English Sheepdog,
Irish Setter, Poodle, Dachshund, Alaskan Malamute,
Schnauzer

Differentiating Blood Loss from Hemolytic Anemia
Blood Loss
Serum or plasma protein concentration normal to low
Clinical evidence of hemorrhage
No icterus, hemoglobinemia, spherocytosis,
hemosiderinuria, autoagglutination, splenomegaly,
or red blood cell (RBC) changes
Negative direct Coombs test

Hemolysis
Serum or plasma protein concentration normal to high
Rarely clinical evidence of hemorrhage
Icterus common
Hemoglobinuria/hemoglobinemia
Spherocytosis
Hemosiderinuria
Autoagglutination sometimes seen
Direct Coombs test usually positive
Splenomegaly
RBC changes numerous

Nonregenerative Anemia

Differential Diagnosis

Anemia of Chronic Disease

Erythropoietin-Related Conditions
Renal disease
Hypothyroidism
Hypoadrenocorticism
Panhypopituitarism
Growth hormone deficiency
Reduced oxygen requirement
Increased oxygen release

Iron Deficiency Anemia
Chronic inflammation
Chronic hemorrhage
Dietary iron deficiency

Marrow Disorders

Toxic Red Cell Aplasia
Estrogen related
Phenylbutazone related
Other drugs

Hyperestrogenism (Iatrogenic, Neoplastic)

Infection
Feline leukemia virus (FeLV)
Feline immunodeficiency virus (FIV)
Parvovirus
Ehrlichiosis
Babesiosis
Mycoplasma haemofelis
Endotoxemia

Immunotherapy

Myelofibrosis
Feline leukemia virus (FeLV) infection
Pyruvate kinase deficiency anemia
Idiopathic

Myelophthisic Disease
Acute leukemias
Chronic leukemias
Multiple myeloma
Lymphoma
Systemic mast cell disease Malignant histiocytosis
Metastatic carcinoma
Histoplasmosis

Myelodysplasia
    Idiopathic
    FeLV/FIV
    Preleukemic syndrome

Pure Red Cell Aplasia

Ineffective Erythropoiesis
  Macrocytic (rare)
    Intrinsic marrow disease
    Vitamin B_{12} deficiency
    Folic acid deficiency

  Normocytic
    Myelofibrosis
    Intrinsic erythroid disease

  Microcytic
    Iron deficiency
    Globin or porphyrin deficiency

  Time Related
    Hemolysis or hemorrhage (during the first 3-5 days)

Diagnosis

Nonregenerative Anemias without Other Cytopenias
Examine bone marrow.

  Severe Erythroid Hypoplasia
    Pure red cell aplasia

  Normal to Mild Erythroid Hypoplasia
    Inflammatory disease
    Renal disease
    Neoplasia
    Hepatic disease
    Hypothyroidism
    Hypoadrenocorticism

  Hypercellular Bone Marrow
    Less than 30% blast forms: consider
      myelodysplastic syndrome
    Greater than 30% blast forms: consider
      hemopoietic neoplasia

*Nonregenerative Anemias with Leukopenia and/or
Thrombocytopenia*
Examine bone marrow.

  Panhypoplasia
    Aplastic anemia

Disease Determined by Core Biopsy
Myelonecrosis
Myelofibrosis

Hypercellular Bone Marrow
Less than 30% blast forms: myelodysplastic syndrome
More than 30% blast forms: hemopoietic neoplasia

Regenerative Anemia

Differential Diagnosis

Hemolysis
Immune mediated
- Intravascular
- Extravascular

Blood Loss Anemia
Trauma
Coagulopathy
- Clotting factor deficiency
- Disseminated intravascular coagulation (DIC)
- Platelet disorders
- Anticoagulant rodenticides
Endoparasites
GI blood loss
Severe ectoparasites (fleas)

Oxidative Injury (Heinz Body)
Onion ingestion
Acetaminophen (cats)
Zinc ingestion (pennies minted after 1982, zinc oxide ointment, zinc-plated bolts and screws)
Benzocaine ingestion (dogs)
D-L Methionine (cats)
Phenolic compounds (mothballs)
Phenazopyridine (cats)

Erythrocytic Parasites
Haemobartonella spp.
Babesia spp.
Cytauxzoon spp.

Fragmentation (Microangiopathic)
Disseminated intravascular coagulation (DIC)
Heartworm disease
Hemangiosarcoma
Vasculitis
Hemolytic-uremic syndrome
Diabetes mellitus

Other

Copper toxicity
Neonatal isoerythrolysis
Hereditary nonspherocytic hemolytic anemia
Pyruvate kinase deficiency
Feline porphyria
Hemolysis in Abyssinian and Somali cats

Coagulopathies, Inherited and Acquired

Differential Diagnosis

Inherited Clotting Factor Deficiencies

Hemophilia A (factor VIII deficiency)
Hemophilia B (factor IX deficiency)
Factor XII deficiency (Hageman trait) (Miniature and Standard Poodle, Shar-Pei, German Shorthair Pointer, cats)
Vitamin K–dependent factor deficiency: factors II, VII, IX, X (Devon Rex cats)
Factor I: hypofibrinogenemia or dysfibrinogenemia (St. Bernard, Borzoi)
Factor II: hypoprothrombinemia (Boxer, Otterhound, English Cocker Spaniel)
Factor VII: hypoproconvertinemia (Beagle, Malamute, Boxer, Bulldog, Miniature Schnauzer)
Factor X deficiency (Cocker Spaniel, Parson Russell Terrier)
Hemophilia C (factor XI deficiency: English Springer Spaniel, Great Pyrenees, Kerry Blue Terrier)
Prekallikrein deficiency (Fletcher factor)

Acquired Clotting Factor Deficiency

Liver disease
• Decreased clotting factor production
• Qualitative disorders
Cholestasis
Vitamin K antagonists
Autoimmune disease (lupus anticoagulant)
Disseminated intravascular coagulation (DIC)
Neoplasia

Clinical Manifestations of Primary and Secondary Hemostatic Defects

Primary Hemostatic Defects

Thrombocytopenia and diseases that cause platelet dysfunction such as uremia, von Willebrand disease, monoclonal gammopathies,

and vector-borne diseases)—typically see manifestations of superficial bleeding
- Petechiae, ecchymoses
- Bleeding from mucosal surfaces (e.g., bleeding from gingiva, melena, hematochezia, epistaxis, hematuria)
- Bleeding in skin
- Hematomas rare
- Prolonged bleeding immediately after venipuncture

Secondary Hemostatic Defects

Clotting factor deficiencies, rodenticide poisoning, liver disease—typically see manifestations of deep bleeding
- Petechiae, ecchymoses rare
- Hematomas common
- Bleeding into body cavities, joints, muscles
- Delayed bleeding after venipuncture

Expected Hemostatic Test Results in Selected Diseases

- Thrombocytopenia—increased buccal mucosal bleeding time (BMBT), decreased platelet count (PLT), normal activated partial thromboplastin time (APTT), normal prothrombin time (PT), normal fibrin degradation products (FDP)
- Platelet dysfunction (e.g., aspirin treatment)—increased BMBT, normal PLT, increased APTT, normal, PT, normal FDP
- Intrinsic pathway defect (e.g., hemophilia A or B)—normal BMBT, normal PLT, increased APTT, normal PT, normal FDP
- Factor VII deficiency—normal BMBT, normal PLT, normal APTT, increased PT, normal, FDP
- Multiple factor defects (e.g., vitamin K antagonism)—normal BMBT, normal PLT, increased APTT, increased PT, normal FDP
- Common pathway defect (e.g., factor X deficiency)—normal BMBT, normal PLT, increased APTT, increased PT, normal FDP
- Disseminated intravascular coagulation (DIC) —increased BMBT, decreased PLT, increased APTT, increased PT, increased FDP
- von Willebrand disease—increased BMBT, normal PLT, normal APTT, normal PT, normal FDP

Leukocyte Disorders

Differential Diagnosis

Pelger-Huët anomaly (many breeds of dogs and cats)
• Neutrophil function not altered
Chédiak-Higashi syndrome (blue smoke-colored Persian cats)
Canine leukocyte adhesion deficiency: fatal defect (Irish Setter and Irish Setter crosses)
Cyclic hemopoiesis (cyclic neutropenia): fatal defect (gray Collies)
Birman cat neutrophil granulation anomaly: neutrophil function not altered
Hypereosinophilic syndrome (cats): may eventually be fatal
Severe combined immunodeficiency of Parson Russell Terriers: fatal defect
Canine X-linked severe combined immunodeficiency: fatal defect (many breeds)
Defective neutrophil function in Doberman Pinscher: need frequent antimicrobial therapy
Immunodeficiency of Shar-Peis
Immunodeficiency of Weimaraners
Lysosomal storage diseases (many types described, all rare, many breeds)

Platelet Dysfunction

Differential Diagnosis

Acquired Platelet Dysfunction

Drugs
Prostaglandin inhibitors (NSAIDs)
Vaccines
Antibiotics
Antifungals
Phenothiazines
Aminophylline
Diltiazem
Isoproterenol

Secondary to Disease
Renal disease
Liver disease
Myeloproliferative disorders

Systemic lupus erythematosus (SLE)
Dysproteinemias

Hereditary
von Willebrand disease (many breeds)
Canine thrombopathia (Basset Hound, Foxhound, Spitz)
Canine thrombasthenic thrombopathia (Otterhound, Great Pyrenees)
Collagen deficiency diseases/Ehler-Danlos syndrome (many breeds)

Splenitis/Splenomegaly

Differential Diagnosis for Splenomegaly

Splenic Mass (Asymmetric Splenomegaly)
Nodular hyperplasia (lymphoid, fibrohistiocytic)
Hematoma
Neoplasia
- Hemangiosarcoma
- Hemangioma
- Leiomyosarcoma
- Fibrosarcoma
- Histiocytic sarcoma
- Leiomyoma
- Myelolipoma
- Metastatic disease

Abscess
Extramedullary hematopoiesis
Granuloma

Uniform Splenomegaly
Congestion
Drugs
Portal hypertension
Right-sided heart failure
Splenic torsion

Hyperplasia
Chronic infection
Inflammatory bowel disease
Systemic lupus erythematosus (SLE)
Polycythemia vera

Extramedullary Hematopoiesis
Chronic anemia
Immune-mediated hemolytic anemia
Immune-mediated thrombocytopenia

Neoplasia
Lymphoma
Systemic mastocytosis
Primary mast cell tumor
Metastatic neoplasia
Multiple myeloma
Acute and chronic leukemias
Malignant histiocytosis
Polycythemia vera

Nonneoplastic Infiltrative Disease
Amyloidosis
Hypereosinophilic syndrome (cats)

Inflammation
Suppurative
Sepsis
Bacterial endocarditis
Infectious canine hepatitis
Foreign body
Penetrating wounds
Toxoplasmosis

Granulomatous
Cryptococcosis
Histoplasmosis
Mycobacteriosis
Leishmaniasis

Pyogranulomatous
Feline infectious peritonitis (FIP)
Blastomycosis
Sporotrichosis

Eosinophilic
Eosinophilic gastroenteritis
Hypereosinophilic syndrome
Neoplasia

Lymphoplasmacytic
Ehrlichiosis
Hemotropic mycoplasmosis
Lymphoplasmacytic enteritis
Pyometra
Brucellosis
Anaplasmosis

Necrotic Tissue
Torsion
Necrotic center of neoplasms

Infectious canine hepatitis
Anaerobic infection
Systemic calicivirosis
Tularemia
Salmonellosis

Infectious Causes

Viral

Feline leukemia virus (FeLV)
Feline immunodeficiency virus (FIV)
Feline infectious peritonitis (FIP)
Infectious canine hepatitis

Bacterial

Canine brucellosis
Mycoplasmosis
Borreliosis
Plague
Tularemia
Streptococcosis
Staphylococcosis
Salmonellosis
Francisella infection
Endotoxemia

Fungal

Cryptococcosis
Histoplasmosis
Blastomycosis

Rickettsial

Ehrlichiosis
Rocky Mountain spotted fever
Q fever *(Coxiella burnetii)*
Mycoplasma haemofelis

Protozoal

Toxoplasmosis
Cytauxzoonosis (cat)
Babesiosis (*Babesia canis* and *B. gibsoni*)
Leishmaniasis (dog)

Thrombocytopenia

Differential Diagnosis

Increased Platelet Destruction/Sequestration/Utilization
Immune-mediated thrombocytopenia
Drug-induced thrombocytopenia

Infectious (*Anaplasma* spp., *Bartonella* spp., sepsis)
Microangiopathy
Disseminated intravascular coagulation
Neoplasia (immune-mediated, microangiography)
Live viral vaccine–induced thrombocytopenia
Hemolytic uremic syndrome/thrombotic thrombocytopenic
 purpura
Vasculitis
Splenomegaly
Splenic torsion
Endotoxemia
Acute hepatic necrosis
Hemorrhage

Decreased Platelet Production
Drug-induced megakaryocytic hypoplasia (estrogen,
 phenylbutazone, melphalan, lomustine, β-lactams)
Myelophthisis
Idiopathic bone marrow aplasia
Retroviral infection (FeLV/FIV)
Immune-mediated megakaryocytic hypoplasia
Cyclic thrombocytopenia
Idiopathic bone marrow aplasia
Ehrlichiosis

Immunologic and Immune-Mediated Disorders

Autoimmune Skin Diseases
Immune-Mediated Disease
Immune System Components
Mechanisms of Immunopathologic Injury
Organ Systems Affected by Autoimmune Disorders in the Dog and Cat
Systemic Lupus Erythematosus (SLE)

Autoimmune Skin Diseases

Differential Diagnosis

Generalized Pustular/Crusting Dermatosis

Pemphigus foliaceus (PF) (nose, ear pinna, and footpad typically affected)

Superficial pustular drug reactions (nasal and footpad lesions may be absent)

Others: rare presentation—systemic lupus erythematosus (SLE), sterile eosinophilic pustulosis, linear immunoglobulin A (IgA) pustular dermatosis, subcorneal pustular dermatosis

Focal Pustular/Crusting Dermatosis

Face, footpads: PF

Face and ears only: PF (early), pemphigus erythematosus (PE), drug eruptions, lupus erythematosus

Nasal only: discoid lupus erythematosus (DLE), PF (early), PE

Mucocutaneous and Mucosal Ulcerations

Pemphigus vulgaris (may also have oral lesions)

Mucous membrane bullous pemphigoid

Epidermolysis bullosa acquisita

Erythema multiforme (target lesions, cutaneous lesions)

Bullous SLE

Drug reactions

Linear IgA bullous dermatosis, toxic epidermal necrolysis (rare)

Nonmucosal Ulcerations (Axillae, Inguinae, Pinnae, Other Haired Areas)

Bullous pemphigoid

Epidermolysis bullosa acquisita
Linear IgA bullous dermatosis
Bullous SLE
Canine vesicular cutaneous lupus erythematosus (idiopathic
  ulcerative dermatosis of Collies, Shetland Sheepdogs)
Erythema multiforme (EM)
Toxic epidermal necrolysis
Drug eruptions
Pemphigus vulgaris

Depigmenting Skin Diseases

Nasal only: DLE, vitiligo-like syndrome,
  uveodermatologic syndrome, early PF or PE
Nose, footpad, lip, eyelid, mucocutaneous area:
  uveodermatologic syndrome (uveitis also)
Haircoat or skin: idiopathic leukotrichia or leukoderma

Miscellaneous

Focal alopecia: alopecia areata, rabies vaccine, focal
  vasculitis
Widespread noninflammatory alopecia: alopecia areata,
  pseudopelade
Erythematous target lesions: erythema multiforme
Nodular ulcerative lesions: nodular panniculitis
Purpura, hemorrhage, punched-out lesions
Ear margin necrosis, dependent edema: vasculitis,
  proliferative necrotizing otitis of kittens, cryoglobulinemia
  and cryofibrinogenemia, proliferative thrombovascular
  necrosis of the pinnae

Immune-Mediated Disease

Laboratory Diagnosis

Direct Coombs Test
Immune-mediated hemolytic anemia
Hemolytic anemia in systemic lupus erythematosus (SLE)

Antiplatelet Antibodies
Immune-mediated thrombocytopenia

Antineutrophil Antibodies
Immune-mediated neutropenia

Thyroxin and Thyroglobulin Autoantibodies
Hypothyroidism

Acetylcholine Receptor Autoantibodies
Myasthenia gravis

2M Myofiber Autoantibodies
Masticatory muscle myositis

Antinuclear Antibody
SLE
Chronic antigenic stimulation

Rheumatoid Factor
Rheumatoid arthritis (RA)

Direct Immunofluorescence
Antibody-complement deposition

Differential Diagnosis for Immune-Mediated Arthritis

Erosive Immune-Mediated Arthritides
RA (dog, rarely in cat)
Periosteal proliferative polyarthritis (cat, rarely in dog)

Nonerosive Immune-Mediated Arthritides
Idiopathic polyarthritis
- **Type I:** uncomplicated idiopathic arthritis (most common)
- **Type II:** idiopathic arthritis associated with infection remote from joints—respiratory tract, tonsils, conjunctiva (chlamydia in cats), urinary tract, uterus, skin, oral cavity
- **Type III:** idiopathic arthritis associated with gastroenteritis
- **Type IV:** idiopathic arthritis associated with malignant neoplasia—squamous cell carcinoma, heart base tumor, leiomyoma, mammary carcinoma, myeloproliferative disease (cats)

SLE
Drug-induced polyarthritis
- Sulfas, lincomycin, erythromycin, cephalosporins, penicillins, trimethoprim-sulfa (especially Doberman Pinscher)

Vaccination reaction
Polyarthritis/polymyositis syndrome
Polyarthritis/meningitis syndrome
Familial renal amyloidosis in Chinese Shar-Peis
Polyarthritis in adolescent Akitas
Polyarthritis nodosa (inflammatory condition of small arteries—histopathologic diagnosis)

Immune System Components

Function

Humoral immunity

B Lymphocytes and Plasma Cells
Production of immunoglobulins

Cellular Immunity

T Lymphocytes
Production of lymphokines
Helper T cells
- Stimulate immune reactivity
Suppressor T cells
- Suppress immune reactivity
Antibody-dependent cell-mediated cytotoxicity
Natural killer cells
- Direct cytotoxicity

Phagocytic Cells

Mononuclear Phagocytic Cells
Antigen presentation
Phagocytosis of particles

Neutrophils and Eosinophils
Phagocytosis of particles
Antibody-dependent cell-mediated cytotoxicity

Mechanisms of Immunopathologic Injury

Type I (immediate)
- Humoral immune system (T-helper cells and B cells), IgE, mast cells, inflammatory mediators)
- Skin, respiratory tract, GI tract commonly affected
- Examples include acute anaphylactic reaction, atopy, allergic bronchitis, feline asthma

Type II (cytotoxic)
- Humoral immune system (IgG and IgM)
- Hematologic systems, neuromuscular junctions, and skin commonly affected
- Examples include immune-mediated hemolytic anemia, immune-mediated thrombocytopenia, myasthenia gravis, pemphigus foliaceous

Type III (immune complex)
- Soluble immune complexes
- Kidney, joints, and skin commonly affected
- Examples include glomerulonephritis, systemic lupus erythematosus, rheumatoid arthritis

Type IV (delayed type)
- Sensitized T lymphocytes, cytokines, neutrophils, and macrophages
- Endocrine glands, muscle commonly affected
- Examples include lymphocytic thyroiditis, myositis

Organ Systems Affected by Autoimmune Disorders in the Dog and Cat

Differential Diagnosis

Hematologic
- Immune-mediated hemolytic anemia
- Pure red cell aplasia
- Immune-mediated thrombocytopenia
- Idiopathic neutropenia

Joints (*see* Differential Diagnosis for Immune-Mediated Arthritis)

Skin (*see* Autoimmune Skin Diseases)

Eye
- Uveitis
- Retinitis

Kidney
- Glomerulonephritis

Respiratory Tract
- Allergic rhinitis
- Allergic bronchitis (asthma)
- Pulmonary infiltrates with eosinophils

Gastrointestinal Tract
- Feline stomatitis, gingivitis
- Lymphocytic, plasmacytic enteritis
- Anal furunculosis (perianal fistula)

Neurologic System
- Myasthenia gravis
- Myositis
- Polyradiculoneuritis
- Granulomatous meningoencephalitis
- Polyarteritis

Endocrine Glands
- Thyroiditis (hypothyroidism)
- Adrenalitis (hypoadrenocorticism)
- Insulitis (diabetes mellitus)

Multisystemic Immune Disease
- Systemic lupus erythematosus

Systemic Lupus Erythematosus (SLE)

Organs and Tissues Affected

Red blood cells
- Immune-mediated hemolytic anemia
- Pure red cell aplasia

Platelets
- Immune-mediated thrombocytopenia

Glomeruli
- Glomerulonephritis

Synovium
- Nonerosive polyarthritis

Blood vessels
- Vasculitis

Epidermis
- Dermatitis

Neutrophils
- Immune-mediated neutrophilia

Clotting factors
- Coagulopathy

Central nervous system
- Seizures, focal signs

Skeletal muscle/nerve end plate
- Polymyositis
- Polyneuritis
- Myasthenia gravis

Criteria for Diagnosis in Dogs and Cats

SLE is diagnosed when three or more of the following criteria are manifested simultaneously or at any time:

Antinuclear antibodies (ANAs)
- Abnormal ANA titer in the absence of drugs or infectious or neoplastic conditions known to be associated with abnormal titers

Cutaneous lesions
- Depigmentation, erythema, erosions, ulcerations, crusts, scaling, with biopsy findings consistent with SLE

Oral ulcers
- Oral or nasopharyngeal ulceration, usually painless

Arthritis
- Nonerosive, nonseptic arthritis involving two or more peripheral joints

Renal disorders
- Glomerulonephritis or persistent proteinuria in the absence of urinary tract infection

Anemia/thrombocytopenia
- Hemolytic anemia/thrombocytopenia in the absence of offending drugs

Leukopenia
- Low total white cell count

Polymyositis or myocarditis
- Inflammatory disease of skeletal or cardiac muscles

Serositis
- Presence of a nonseptic inflammatory cavity effusion (abdominal, pleural, or pericardial)

Neurologic disorders
- Seizures or psychosis in the absence of known disorders

Antiphospholipids
- Prolongation of activated partial thromboplastin time (APTT) that fails to correct with a 1:1 mixture of patient's and normal plasma, in the absence of heparin or fibrin degradation products (FDPs)

Infectious Disease

Anaplasmosis, Canine

Clinical Signs

Infection may be subclinical
Fever
Depression
Inappetence
Scleral injection
Lameness, stiffness, reluctance to move
Coughing (soft and nonproductive)
Lymphadenopathy
Splenomegaly
Neutrophilic polyarthritis (rare)
CNS signs?
Vomiting/diarrhea
May be more susceptible to other infections

Laboratory Abnormalities

Thrombocytopenia
Lymphopenia
Eosinopenia
Mild regenerative anemia
Hypoalbuminemia
Mild to moderately elevated hepatic enzymes

Bacterial Infections, Systemic

Differential Diagnosis

Leptospirosis

Hepatic dysfunction, renal dysfunction, fever, anterior uveitis, icterus

Coagulation abnormalities, vomiting/diarrhea, icterus, polyuria/polydipsia, anorexia

Some cases may be subclinical

Borreliosis (Lyme Disease)

Fever, inappetence/lethargy, lymphadenopathy, polyarthritis

Glomerulonephritis/acute, progressive renal failure, mild dermatologic lesions

Meningitis/encephalitis (rare), myocarditis

Mycobacteriosis

Often asymptomatic, skin lesions, dermal nodules, draining tracts, lymphadenopathy, bronchopneumonia, pulmonary nodules, hilar lymphadenopathy, vomiting, diarrhea secondary to intestinal malabsorption, feline leprosy

Brucellosis (Dogs)

Clinical signs may be mild to absent

Fever, lymphadenopathy

Epididymitis, scrotal enlargement, scrotal dermatitis, infertility in males

Abortion, early embryonic death, fetal resorption, in pregnant bitches

Discospondylitis

Rarely uveitis, glomerulonephritis, meningoencephalitis

Tetanus

Localized tetanus, especially cats; stiffness in a muscle of limb

Generalized tetanus stiff gait, outstretched or dorsally curved tails, extreme muscle rigidity, hypersensitivity to touch, light, and sounds

Ears erect, lips drawn back (sardonic grin), protrusion of globe, enophthalmos

Trismus (lockjaw), laryngeal spasm, regurgitation, megaesophagus leading to aspiration pneumonia, seizures

Botulism

Generalized lower motor neuron and parasympathetic dysfunction, cranial nerve signs, mentation is normal
Quadriplegia, megaesophagus, respiratory paralysis; may lead to death

Feline Plague *(Yersinia pestis)*

Spread by fleas
May show signs of bubonic, septicemic, and pneumonic plague
Depression
Cervical swellings, draining tracts
Dyspnea or cough

Mycoplasmosis/Ureaplasmosis (Cats)

Conjunctivitis, sneezing, mucopurulent nasal discharge, coughing, dyspnea, fever, lameness, swollen joints, subcutaneous abscessation

Members of the Order Rickettsiales of Clinical Importance in Dogs and Cats

Rickettsioses (Spotted Fever Group Rickettsiae)

Rickettsia rickettsii
Species of the following tick genera transmit spotted-fever group agents: *Dermacentor, Rhipicephalus, Haemaphysalis,* and *Amblyomma*

Ehrlichiosis (Canine)

Ehrlichia canis, E. chaffeensis, E. ewingii, E. muris, and *E. ruminantium*

Anaplasmosis (Canine and Feline)

Anaplasma phagocytophilium
Anaplasma platys (canine cyclic thrombocytopenia: mildly pathogenic)

Neorickettsiosis

Neorickettsia helminthoeca, N. risticii

Bartonellosis, Canine

Clinical Findings

- Many species of *Bartonella* are suspected to cause disease in dogs (e.g., *B. vinsonii, B. henselae, B. clarridgeae, B. elizabethae*)
- Fever
- Endocarditis, myocarditis, arrhythmias

- Epistaxis
- Intermittent lameness
- Bone pain
- Granulomatous lymphadenitis
- Dermatologic lesions/cutaneous vasculitis
- Anterior uveitis
- Polyarthritis
- Meningoencephalitis
- Immune-mediated hemolytic anemia
- Thrombocytopenia
- Eosinophilia
- Peliosis hepatitis
- Granulomatous hepatitis
- Chronic weight loss

Bartonellosis, Feline

Subclinical Disease in Most Cats

Uveitis?
Endocarditis?

Anaplasmosis

Anaplasma phagocytophilum, formally known as *Ehrlichia equi,*
E. phagocytophila

Cause of Canine Granulocytic Ehrlichiosis

Clinical Signs
Fever
Depression
Inappetence
Scleral injection
Lameness/polyarthritis
Coughing
Lymphadenopathy
Splenomegaly
Vomiting/diarrhea
Lymphopenia, eosinopenia, mild nonregenerative anemia
Hypoalbuminemia, elevated hepatic enzymes

Anaplasma Platys

Cause of Canine Thrombocytic Anaplasmosis
Forms morula that can be visualized in platelets

Clinical Signs
Majority of cases in United States have been mild or
subclinical

More severe signs in European or South American cases include:
- Fever
- Splenomegaly
- Hemorrhage

Ehrlichiosis, Canine

Clinical Findings

Acute
Fever
Anorexia/weight loss
Depression
Serous or purulent oculonasal discharge
Lymphadenopathy/splenomegaly
Peripheral edema
Petechial and ecchymotic hemorrhages
Neurologic signs (ataxia, seizures, vestibular signs, hyperesthesia, cranial nerve defects)
Dyspnea
History of recent or present tick bite
Thrombocytopenia
Leukopenia followed by leukocytosis and monocytosis
Low-grade nonregenerative anemia, unless hemorrhage
Variable *Ehrlichia* titer, polymerase chain reaction (PCR) positive

Subclinical
No clinical abnormalities apparent
Hyperglobulinemia, thrombocytopenia, neutropenia, lymphocytosis, monocytosis
Positive *Ehrlichia* titer, PCR positive

Chronic
Depression
Pale mucous membranes
Weight loss
Abdominal pain
Splenomegaly
Epistaxis, retinal hemorrhage, petechia and ecchymoses, melena, hematochezia, hematuria, and other examples of hemorrhage
Lymphadenopathy
Stiffness, swollen/painful joints, polymyositis
Hepatomegaly
Dyspnea, interstitial or alveolar lung infiltrates

Perivascular retinitis, hyphema, retinal detachment, anterior uveitis, corneal edema

Seizures, paresis, meningeal pain, cranial nerve deficits

Arrhythmias

Polyuria/polydipsia

Secondary opportunistic infection (viral papillomatosis, protozoal infections, bacteriuria)

Monocytosis, lymphocytosis, thrombocytopenia, nonregenerative anemia, hyperglobulinemia, hypoalbuminemia, hypocellular bone marrow, proteinuria, polyclonal or monoclonal gammopathy, nonseptic suppurative polyarthritis, cerebrospinal fluid (CSF) mononuclear pleocytosis

Increased alanine aminotransferase (ALT) and alkaline phosphatase (ALP)

Positive *Ehrlichia* titer, PCR positive

Influenza, Canine

Clinical Features

- Most outbreaks in group housed dogs (race tracks, animal shelters)
- Individual pets often had a recent history of exposure to other dogs
- Mild form may cause a harsh cough similar to cough heard with infectious tracheobronchitis
- More commonly cough is soft and moist, cough may persist for as long as a month
- Fever
- Mucopurulent nasal discharge
- Increased respiratory rate progressing to respiratory distress
- May progress to overt pneumonia
- Mortality rate less than 5%. Very young and very old are most at risk

Neorickettsiosis Canine

Neorickettsia helminthoeca (salmon poisoning disease)

Restricted to western slopes of Cascade Mountains from northern California to southern Vancouver Island

Vector is a fluke *Nanophyetus salmincola*. Dogs become infected from ingesting parasitized fish.

Clinical Signs

Fever

Anorexia/weight loss

Depression

Lymphadenopathy

Vomiting

Diarrhea

Hematochezia

Neutrophilia with left shift, lymphopenia, monocytosis, thrombocytopenia

Electrolyte derangements, elevated hepatic enzymes, hypoalbuminemia

Neorickettsia risticii

Cause of equine Potomac horse fever

Vector is suspected to be a fluke *Acanthatrium oregonense*

Has been identified by culture and PCR in dogs with the following signs:

Lethargy

Intermittent vomiting

Bleeding tendencies

Polyarthritis

Neurologic signs

Dependent edema

Anemia

Thrombocytopenia

Mycoses, Systemic

Clinical Findings

Blastomycosis

Restricted primarily to Mississippi, Ohio, Missouri, Tennessee, and St. Lawrence River valleys plus the southern Great Lakes and the southern Mid-Atlantic states

Sporting breeds predisposed because of greater exposure, males more than females

Anorexia, depression, weight loss, cachexia, fever, mild to severe dyspnea, cyanosis, cough, chylothorax, diffuse lymphadenopathy, papules, plaques and ulcerative nodules, paronychia, chorioretinitis, conjunctivitis, keratitis, iridocyclitis, anterior uveitis, subretinal granulomas, retinal detachment, secondary glaucoma, lameness from osteomyelitis, splenomegaly

Radiographically, infiltrative bronchointerstitial and alveolar disease, hilar lymphadenopathy

Histoplasmosis

Restricted primarily to Mississippi, Missouri, and Ohio River valleys and Mid-Atlantic states

Sporting breeds predisposed because of greater exposure

Common clinical signs include anorexia, fever, depression, weight loss, cough, dyspnea, diarrhea (large bowel diarrhea most often, may see protein-losing enteropathy), hepatosplenomegaly, icterus, ascites, and lymphadenopathy.

Less common signs include lameness secondary to osteo-myelitis or polyarthritis, chorioretinitis, central nervous system (CNS) disease, and cutaneous lesions.

Differential Diagnosis for Gastrointestinal Signs Seen in Dogs and Cats with Histoplasmosis

Large Intestinal Disease
Diet-Associated Colitis
- Dietary hypersensitivity
- Foreign material–induced colitis

Idiopathic Colitis
- Lymphocytic-plasmacytic colitis
- Eosinophilic colitis
- Granulomatous colitis
- Histiocytic ulcerative colitis of Boxer dogs
- Suppurative colitis

Parasitic and Protozoal Colitis
- Trichuriasis (whipworm)
- Ancylostomiasis (hookworm)
- Entamebiasis
- Balantidiasis
- Giardiasis

Bacterial colitis
- Salmonellosis
- Campylobacter jejuni
- Yersinia enterocolitica, Y. pseudotuberculosis
- Mycobacteria
- Clostridium perfringens, C. difficile

Fungal colitis
- Candidiasis
- GI pythiosis
- Prototheocosis

Cecocolic or ileocolic intussusception
Pancreatitis-associated colitis

Small Intestinal Disease
Idiopathic inflammatory bowel disease
- Lymphocytic-plasmacytic enteritis
- Eosinophilic enteritis
- Granulomatous enteritis

Intestinal lymphosarcoma
Parasitic enteritis
- Ancylostomiasis
- Toxocariasis
- Chronic giardiasis

Infectious enteritis
- Small intestinal bacterial overgrowth
- GI pythiosis

Lymphangiectasia

Exocrine pancreatic insufficiency

Partial intestinal obstruction

Chronic enteropathy of Shar-Peis

Immunoproliferative enteritis of Basenjis

Coccidioidomycosis

Primarily southwestern United States, California, Mexico, Central and South America

Common clinical signs include lameness with swollen and painful joints and bones, cough, dyspnea, anorexia, weakness, pleural effusion, and cutaneous lesions over infected bones.

Less common signs include myocarditis, icterus, renomegaly, splenomegaly, hepatomegaly, orchitis, epididymitis, keratitis, iritis, granulomatous uveitis, glaucoma, seizures, ataxia, and central vestibular disease.

Cryptococcosis

Found worldwide, more common in southern United States, most common in cats

Common clinical signs include upper respiratory signs, unilateral to bilateral nasal discharge, soft masses in nasal cavity or over bridge of nose, ulcerative skin lesions, lymphadenopathy, granulomatous chorioretinitis, and retinal detachment.

Less common signs include fever, lung involvement, CNS involvement caused by invasion through cribriform plate, depression, seizures, circling, ataxia, blindness, head pressing, and paresis.

Aspergillosis

Dogs affected more often than cats

Nasal turbinate destruction, frontal sinus osteomyelitis, mucoid to hemorrhagic nasal discharge, epistaxis

May lead to masticatory muscle atrophy and CNS disease by erosion through cribriform plate

In rare cases, disseminates and causes multiple-organ disease

Pythiosis, Lagenidiosis (Pythium insidiosum, Lagenidium giganteum)

Severe, often fatal, chronic gastrointestinal and cutaneous diseases

Zygomycosis (Multiple Fungi in Class Zygomycetes)

Nasopharyngeal involvement, poorly responsive to therapy

Differential Diagnosis for Systemic Manifestations

Multisystemic granulomatous, neoplastic, and immune-mediated diseases must be differentiated from disseminated systemic mycoses.

Differential Diagnosis for Nodular Skin Disease

Bacteria Skin Disease
- Actinomycosis
- Mycobacteriosis
- Botryomycosis
- Brucellosis
- *Rhodococcus equi* infection
- *Bartonella vinsonii* subsp. *Berkhoffi* infection

Mycotic and Miscellaneous Infectious Skin Disease
- Cryptococcosis
- Blastomycosis
- Coccidioidomycosis
- Sporotrichosis
- Basidiobolomycosis
- Conidiobolomycosis
- Phaeohyphomycosis
- Hyalohyphomycosis
- Eumycotic mycetoma
- Dermatophytic mycetoma
- Protothecosis
- Pythiosis
- Lagenidiosis
- Nodular leishmaniasis

Noninfectious Pyogranulomatous Skin Disease
- Foreign body reaction
- Idiopathic nodular panniculitis
- Sebaceous adenitis (nodular form)
- Canine cutaneous sterile pyogranulomatous/ granuloma syndrome

Neoplasia
- Squamous cell carcinoma
- Cutaneous lymphoma
- Mycosis fungoides (cutaneous T-cell lymphoma)
- Cutaneous histiocytosis

Miscellaneous Diseases
- Systemic lupus erythematosus
- Systemic vasculitis
- Cutaneous embolic disease

Differential Diagnosis for Chorioretinitis, Exudative Retinal Detachment, and Panophthalmitis

Fungal
- Blastomycosis
- Cryptococcosis
- Coccidioidomycosis
- Geotrichosis
- Histoplasmosis
- Aspergillosis

Neoplasia
- Lymphosarcoma
- Metastatic neoplasia

Miscellaneous Infectious Causes
- Protothecosis
- Brucellosis
- Toxoplasmosis
- *Neosporum caninum* infection
- Leishmaniasis
  Lymphadenopathy must be differentiated from numerous causes including lymphosarcoma, other fungal infections, rickettsial diseases, brucellosis, mycobacteriosis, protothecosis, and leishmaniasis.
  Solitary bone lesions must be differentiated from primary or metastatic neoplasia and other fungal or bacterial osteomyelitis.

Polysystemic Protozoal Diseases

Clinical Findings

Feline Toxoplasmosis
Acute toxoplasmosis: may induce a self-limiting, small bowel diarrhea

Disseminated toxoplasmosis: overwhelming intracellular replication of tachyzoites after primary infection—depression, anorexia, fever, hypothermia, peritoneal effusion, icterus, dyspnea, death—coinfection with feline leukemia virus (FeLV), feline immunodeficiency virus (FIV), feline infectious peritonitis (FIP), and others may predispose to disseminated toxoplasmosis

Chronic toxoplasmosis: anterior or posterior uveitis, fever, muscle hyperesthesia, weight loss, anorexia, seizures, ataxia, icterus, diarrhea, pancreatitis

Canine Toxoplasmosis

Respiratory, gastrointestinal, neuromuscular signs: fever, vomiting, diarrhea, dyspnea, icterus, ataxia, seizures, tremors, cranial nerve deficits, paresis, paralysis, myositis, lower motor neuron disease, myocardial disease, chorioretinitis, anterior uveitis, iridocyclitis, optic neuritis (ocular lesions less common in dogs than cats)

Neosporosis

Most common in neonates but can be seen at any age

Ascending paralysis, hyperextension of hind limbs, muscle atrophy, polymyositis, multifocal CNS disease, myocarditis, dysphagia, ulcerative dermatitis, pneumonia, hepatitis

Babesiosis

Anemia, fever, pale mucous membranes, tachycardia, tachypnea, depression, anorexia, weakness, icterus, petechiae, hepatosplenomegaly, disseminated intravascular coagulation (DIC), metabolic acidosis, renal disease

Cytauxzoonosis

Fever, anorexia, dyspnea (pneumonitis), depression, icterus, pale mucous membranes, death

Hepatozoonosis (*Hepatozoon canis* and *H. americanum*)

Most common in puppies and immunosuppressed dogs, but *H. americanum* can be primary

Fever, weight loss, severe hyperesthesia, anorexia, anemia, depression, oculonasal discharge, bloody diarrhea

Leishmaniasis

Weight loss, normal to increased appetite, polyuria/polydipsia, muscle wasting, depression, vomiting, diarrhea, cough, epistaxis, sneezing, melena, splenomegaly, facial alopecia, rhinitis, dermatitis, icterus, swollen and painful joints, uveitis, conjunctivitis

Dermatologic lesions include hyperkeratosis, scaling, mucocutaneous ulcers, and intradermal nodules on muzzle, ears, and footpads.

American Trypanosomiasis *(Trypanosoma cruzi)*

Acute infection: myocarditis, heart failure—lymphadenopathy, pale mucous membranes, tachycardia, pulse deficits, hepatomegaly, abdominal distension, anorexia, diarrhea, neurologic signs

Chronic infection: Those that survive acute infection may present with chronic dilative cardiomyopathy—right-sided heart failure, conductive disturbances, supraventricular arrhythmias.

Rocky Mountain Spotted Fever

Clinical Findings

Depression/lethargy
Fever
Anorexia
Myalgia/arthralgia
Lymphadenopathy
Vestibular deficits
Conjunctivitis/scleral congestion/hyphema/iridal and retinal
  hemorrhage
Pneumonitis/dyspnea/cough
Abdominal pain
Edema of face and extremities
Epistaxis
Melena
Hematuria
Anterior uveitis
Rash/petechiae
Nausea/vomiting
Diarrhea
Vasculitis/thrombocytopenia/disseminated intravascular
  coagulation (DIC)
Hyperesthesia/spinal cord signs
Seizures
Cardiac arrhythmias
Icterus
Acute renal failure
Coma/stupor
Polyuria/polydipsia

Sepsis and Systemic Inflammatory Response Syndrome (SIRS)

Definitions

Bacteremia: the presence of viable bacteria in the
  bloodstream
Sepsis: infection-induced systemic inflammation
Severe sepsis: organ dysfunction and manifestations of
  hypoperfusion or hypotension secondary to sepsis
Septic shock: hypotension secondary to sepsis, not responsive
  to intravenous (IV) fluid therapy
SIRS: systemic inflammation caused by either infectious
  or noninfectious processes. Diagnosis of SIRS is based on
  fulfillment of at least two of four criteria (tachycardia,

tachypnea, hypothermia, or hyperthermia and either
leucocytosis, leucopenia, or bands)

Multiple organ dysfunction syndrome (MODS): altered
function of two or more organs secondary to SIRS
such that homeostasis cannot be maintained without
intervention

Acute respiratory distress syndrome (ARDS): a pulmonary
inflammatory disorder characterized by noncardiogenic
pulmonary edema, neutrophilic inflammation, and
hypoxemia

Noninfectious Causes of SIRS

Pancreatitis
Tissue trauma
Heat stroke
Ischemia
Burns
Pansystemic neoplasia

Infectious Causes of SIRS (Sepsis)

Peritonitis
Pyometra
Prostatitis
Prostatic abscess
Pyelonephritis
Pneumonia
Pyothorax
Gastroenteritis
Endocarditis
Nosocomial infections (IV catheters, urinary catheters, etc.)

Clinical Findings of Sepsis and SIRS

Fever or hypothermia
Tachycardia, tachypnea
Neutrophilia with left shift or leukopenia
Anemia
Depression
Bounding or diminished pulses
Brick-red mucus membranes or pallor
Hypothermia
Thrombocytopenia
Hypoalbuminemia, hypoglycemia
Disseminated intravascular coagulation (DIC)
Bilirubinemia
Elevated hepatic enzymes
Azotemia
Oliguria

Lactic acidosis
Hypoxemia
Signs related to underlying condition

Vaccines, Recommended Core vs. Noncore

Core Vaccines for Dogs

- Distemper
- Parvovirus
- Adenovirus-2
- Rabies

Core Vaccines for Cats

- Parvovirus (panleukopenia)
- Herpesvirus-1
- Calicivirus
- Rabies

Noncore Vaccines for Dogs

Need determined by individual clinician after assessment of
   patient risk
- Bordetellosis
- Parainfluenza
- Canine influenza
- Leptospirosis
- Lyme borreliosis
- *Crotalus atrax*
- *Porphyromonas* spp.

Noncore Vaccines for Cats

Need determined by individual clinician after assessment of
   patient risk
- Feline leukemia virus (FeLV)
- Feline immunodeficiency virus (FIV)
- *Chlamydophila felis* (formally, *Chlamydia psittaci*)
- Bordetellosis

Viruses, Canine

Common Viral Agents of Diseases of Dogs

Parvovirus

May be asymptomatic or fulminant disease
Anorexia, lethargy, fever, vomiting, hemorrhagic
   diarrhea, myocarditis (rare)
Worse in very young and parasitized puppies
Neutropenia, hypoalbuminemia, severe dehydration,
   secondary septicemia

Coronavirus

Diarrhea (infrequently blood in feces), vomiting, anorexia, lethargy, often self-limiting

Canine respiratory coronavirus, part of "kennel cough" complex

Coughing, sneezing, nasal discharge

Canine pancytotropic coronavirus

Severe clinical disease in puppies and juvenile dogs

Fever, lethargy, anorexia, vomiting, hemorrhagic diarrhea, ataxia, seizures

Rotavirus

Vomiting, diarrhea (rarely bloody), anorexia, typically recover after 5-7 days

Adenovirus Type 1 (Infectious Canine Hepatitis)

Fever, anorexia, lethargy, depression, abdominal pain, pale mucous membranes, tonsillitis, pharyngitis, coughing, hepatomegaly

Severe cases: coagulation abnormalities, petechiae, ecchymosis, DIC, rarely icterus, hepatic encephalopathy

Anterior uveitis and glomerulonephritis secondary to immune complex deposition

Canine Distemper Virus (*See* the next section)

Canine Influenza A Subtype H3N8 Virus

Acute onset of coughing, sneezing, nasal discharge, ocular discharge

Lowgrade fever

Secondary commensal bacterial infections leading to mucopurulent discharge and productive cough

May lead to pneumonia with high fever, inappetence, productive cough, and increased respiratory effort

Rabies Virus

Variable incubation period, prodromal phase: nervousness, anxiety, paresthesia

Progress to forebrain signs ("furious" form of rabies): irritability, restlessness, pica, photophobia, increased saliva production with decreasing ability to swallow, hyperesthesia progressing to incoordination, seizures, and death

May also progress to "dumb" form: paralysis, lower motor disease, leading to coma, respiratory paralysis, and death

Pseudorabies

Suspected to be result from ingestion of infected raw pork

Neurologic dysfunction: ataxia, abnormal papillary light response, restlessness, trismus, cervical rigidity, ptyalism, tachypnea, excoriation from pruritus of head and neck; vomiting, diarrhea; most dogs die within 48 hours

Parainfluenza and Adenovirus Type 2

Hacking cough with gagging, easily elicited with tracheal palpation; cough may be paroxysmal, usually subsides within 7-10 days, and may lead to secondary bacterial or mycoplasmal infection

Canine Herpesvirus

Abortion, stillbirths; puppies born live progress to crying, hypothermia, soft stools, petechiae, cessation of nursing, and death

Older puppies develop mild respiratory signs that may emerge later as neurologic disease (ataxia, blindness, central vestibular disease).

Adult dogs: usually asymptomatic, rhinitis, pharyngitis, vaginal or preputial hyperemia, hyperplasia of vaginal mucosal lymphoid follicles, submucosal hemorrhage

Canine Oral Papillomavirus

Oral papilloma (warts), may be quite extensive, spontaneously regress

West Nile Virus

Clinical disease is uncommon.

Bornavirus

Seropositivity in the absence of clinical signs appears possible.

Tremors, salivation, mydriasis, circling

Canine Distemper Virus Infection, Clinical Findings

General Signs

Fever
Lethargy
Depression
Anorexia
Dehydration

Respiratory Tract

Mucoid to mucopurulent discharge
Bronchopneumonia
- Coughing
- Crackles on auscultation
- Increased bronchovesicular sounds
- Dyspnea
Sneezing

Gastrointestinal Tract
Vomiting
Small bowel diarrhea

Ocular Disease
Mucopurulent ocular discharge
Chorioretinitis, medallion lesions, optic neuritis, retinal detachment
Keratoconjunctivitis sicca
Anterior uveitis

Neurologic Disease
Spinal cord lesion: paresis and ataxia
Central vestibular disease: head tilt, nystagmus, other cranial nerve and conscious proprioception deficits
Cerebellar disease: ataxia, head bobbing, hypermetria
Cerebral disease: seizures, blindness
Chorea myoclonus: rhythmic jerking of single muscles or muscle groups

Miscellaneous
Tonsillar enlargement
Pustular dermatosis
Hyperkeratosis of nose and footpads
Enamel hypoplasia

In Utero Infection
Stillbirth
Abortion
"Fading puppy" syndrome in neonatal period
Central nervous system signs at birth

Viruses, Feline

American Association of Feline Practitioners Guidelines for Retroviral Testing in Cats

- Sick cats should be tested even if they have tested negative before.
- Cats and kittens should be tested when they are first acquired.
- Even cats not expected to live with other cats should be tested. This provides a health assessment of the individual, other cats may join the household, indoor cats may escape and expose other cats.
- Tests should be performed at adoption and negative cats should be retested a minimum of 60 days later.

- Cats with known recent exposure to a retrovirus-infected cat or a cat with unknown status, particularly via a bite wound, should be tested regardless of previous test results. Testing should be done immediately and, if negative, should be repeated after a minimum of 30 days for FeLV and after a minimum of 60 days for FIV (when the type of potential viral exposure is unknown, retesting for both viruses after 60 days is most practical).
- Cats living in households with other cats infected with FIV or FeLV should be tested annually.
- High-risk cats (cats in cat-dense neighborhoods or cats that fight and get cat-bite wounds and abscesses) should be tested regularly.
- Cats should be tested before initial vaccination against FeLV or FIV.
- Cats used for blood or tissue donation should have negative screening tests for FeLV and FIV and should be negative for real-time PCR tests.
- Intermittent retesting is not necessary for cats with confirmed negative infection status unless there is opportunity for exposure to infected cats or if they become ill.
- Each cat should be individually tested. Testing of one cat as a proxy for another or pooling samples from multiple cats for testing is inappropriate.

Clinical Signs of Rabies Virus Infection in Cats

- Initially signs are nonspecific: lethargy, inappetence, vomiting, diarrhea
- Rapid and continual deterioration of clinical conditions, no waxing and waning
- Behavioral changes: more reclusive or attention-seeking, may unpredictably attack animate, inanimate, or unseen objects
- Irrevocable progression to classic signs, ptyalism with decreased ability to swallow leads to contamination of oral cavity, chin, and forelegs with potentially infectious saliva. Cranial nerve signs such as anisocoria, pupil dysfunction, facial or tongue paresis, and changes in phonation may occur.
- Auditory, visual, or tactile stimulation may elicit profound aggression to self-mutilation.
- Become profoundly moribund to comatose to death. 100% fatal

Feline Infectious Peritonitis (FIP, Feline Coronavirus Infection), Clinical Findings

Signalment and History

Purebred cats from cattery

Multicat households

Younger than 5 years or older than 10 years of age

Previous history of mild, self-limiting gastrointestinal or respiratory disease

Anorexia, weight loss, depression

Seizures, nystagmus, ataxia

Acute, fulminant course in cats with effusive FIP

Chronic, intermittent course in cats with noneffusive FIP

Physical Examination Findings

Fever

Weight loss

Abdominal distension/fluid wave

Abdominal mass (focal intestinal granuloma, lymphadenopathy)

Icterus

Muffled heart or lung sounds

Dyspnea secondary to pleural effusion

Hepatomegaly

Chorioretinitis, iridocyclitis

Splenomegaly

Pale mucous membranes with or without petechiae

Multifocal neurologic abnormalities

Irregularly marginated kidneys

Renomegaly

Clinicopathologic Abnormalities

Complete blood count (CBC): nonregenerative anemia, neutrophilia with or without left shift, lymphopenia

Serum chemistry: elevated alkaline phosphatase (ALP) and alanine aminotransferase (ALT), hyperbilirubinemia, hyperglobulinemia (polyclonal, rarely monoclonal gammopathy), azotemia (prerenal or renal)

Urinalysis: proteinuria

Nonseptic, pyogranulomatous exudate in peritoneal cavity, pleural space, and pericardium

Positive coronavirus antibody titer (especially in noneffusive cases)

Cerebrospinal fluid (CSF) tap: increased protein concentration, neutrophilic pleocytosis, coronavirus antibodies

Histopathology: pyogranulomatous inflammation in perivascular locations of tissues

Positive for coronavirus on immunofluorescence or reverse-transcriptase polymerase chain reaction (RT-PCR) testing of abdominal or pleural effusions (although these tests do not differentiate between FIP-causing viruses and "harmless" feline enteric coronavirus)

Feline Immunodeficiency Virus (FIV) Infection, Clinical Findings

Primary Phase of Infection
Low-grade fever
Lymphadenopathy
Neutropenia

Latent Phase
No clinical signs for months to years

Immunodeficiency Phase

Primary Viral Effects
Weight loss
Nonregenerative anemia, neutropenia, thrombocytopenia
Small bowel diarrhea
Glomerulonephritis
Myeloproliferative disorders
Lymphoma
Renal failure
Anterior uveitis, pars planitis
Behavioral abnormalities

Opportunistic Infectious Agents
Cutaneous: atypical mycobacteriosis, demodicosis, *Notoedres* and *Otodectes* infestation, dermatophytosis, cryptococcosis, cowpox
Gastrointestinal: cryptosporidiosis, coccidiosis, giardiasis, salmonellosis, campylobacteriosis, others
Renal: bacterial infections, FIP, feline leukemia virus (FeLV)
Urinary tract: bacterial infections
Neoplasia: FeLV
Hematologic: *Mycoplasma haemofelis,* FeLV, bartonellosis
Neurologic: toxoplasmosis, cryptococcosis, FIP, FeLV
Ophthalmologic: toxoplasmosis, FIP, cryptococcosis, herpesvirus, bartonellosis
Pneumonia/pneumonitis: bacterial, toxoplasmosis, cryptococcosis

Pyothorax: bacterial
Stomatitis: calicivirus, bacterial, candidiasis, bartonellosis
Upper respiratory: herpesvirus, calicivirus, bacterial, cryptococcosis

Feline Leukemia Virus (FeLV), Clinical Findings

Acute Phase
Fever
Malaise
Diarrhea
Leukopenia

General Signs
Anorexia
Weight loss
Depression
Many FeLV positive cats are asymptomatic at diagnosis

Neoplastic
Lymphoma: mediastinal, multicentric, alimentary, renal
Leukemia: lymphocytic, myelogenous, erythroid, megakaryocytic
Myeloproliferative disorders
Fibrosarcoma

Icterus
Prehepatic: immune-mediated red blood cell (RBC) destruction induced by FeLV or secondary infection with *Mycoplasma haemofelis*
Hepatic: hepatic lymphoma, focal liver necrosis, hepatic lipidosis
Posthepatic: alimentary lymphoma

Bone marrow
Pure red cell aplasia
Regenerative anemia (less common and often associated with coinfection with *Mycoplasma haemofelis*)
Myeloproliferative disease (anemia, leukopenia, thrombocytopenia)

Stomatitis
Bacterial infection
Calicivirus infection

Rhinitis/Pneumonia
Bacteria
Herpesvirus and calicivirus

Renal

Glomerulonephritis

Renal failure

Urinary incontinence: sphincter incompetence or
detrusor hyperactivity

Ocular Lymphoma

Aqueous flare, mass lesions, keratitic precipitates, lens
luxations, glaucoma, anterior uveitis

Neurologic Polyneuropathy or lymphoma

Anisocoria, ataxia, weakness, tetraparesis, paraparesis,
behavioral changes, urinary incontinence

Secondary infection with FIP, *Toxoplasma gondii,
Cryptococcus neoformans*

In Utero Infection

Abortion, stillbirth, infertility, kitten mortality complex
("fading kitten" syndrome)

Lameness

Neutrophilic polyarthritis secondary to immune complex
deposition

Multiple cartilaginous exostoses

Feline Leukemia Virus, Possible Outcomes Following Exposure

Progressive Infection

Viral replication in lymphoid tissue and bone marrow, spread
to mucosal and glandular tissues, leading to shedding of
virus. Most cats become persistently infected and frequently
die of an FeLV-associated disease within a few years.

Regressive Infection

Effective immune response limits viral replication. FeLV
antigen detectable in peripheral blood within 2-3 weeks
after exposure but disappears 2-8 weeks later. May not
ever develop antigenemia. Clinical relevance of regressive
infection is not clear. May have persistent integration of
FeLV DNA in their genome but are unlikely to develop
FeLV-associated diseases. Do not shed virus.

Abortive Exposure

Seen infrequently following experimental FeLV
inoculation characterized by negative results for
culturable virus, antigen, viral RNA, and proviral DNA

Focal Infections

Rare events in which cats have FeLV infection restricted
to certain tissues such as spleen, lymph nodes, small
intestine, or mammary glands.

Other Feline Viral Diseases

Upper Respiratory Tract Viruses

Herpesvirus type 1: ocular and nasal disease

Calicivirus: ocular, nasal, and oral disease; rarely joint disease

Reovirus: Conjunctivitis, respiratory lesions, diarrhea experimentally, no evidence of importance in the field

Enteric Viruses

Feline parvovirus (panleukopenia virus): enteritis, panleukopenia, cerebellar hypoplasia, fetal death

Feline coronavirus: mild enteritis, FIP

Rotavirus: rare cause of mild diarrhea

Astrovirus: uncommon cause of persistent watery diarrhea

Torovirus: may be associated with protruding nictitating membrane and diarrhea syndrome

Miscellaneous

Cowpox virus: mainly see skin lesions; sporadic disease in cats Hantavirus: zoonotic disease of wild rodents; clinical significance in cats not known

Rabies virus

Pseudorabies virus: cats are a rare host, severe behavioral changes, pruritus, paralysis, coma, death

Feline herpesvirus type 2: possible association with feline idiopathic lower urinary tract disease

Joint and Bone Disorders

Arthritis
Bone Disorders

Arthritis

Differential Diagnosis: Infectious Arthritis

Septic Arthritis

Bacterial Suppurative Arthritis
Penetrating wounds
- Animal bites

Iatrogenic
- Infection during surgery, arthrocentesis

Trauma (e.g., hit by car)
Hematogenous
- Endocarditis
- Omphalophlebitis
- Pyoderma
- Other foci of infection

Lyme Arthritis

Borrelia burgdorferi
Transmitted by *Ixodes* ticks

Bacterial L-Form Arthritis

Cell wall–deficient bacteria
Causes suppurative arthritis and subcutaneous abscesses
    in cats

Mycoplasma Arthritis

Debilitated and immunosuppressed animals
M. gatae, M. felis in cats

Fungal Arthritis (Rare)

Coccidioides immitis
Blastomyces dermatitidis
Cryptococcusneoformans
Sporothrix schenckii
Aspergillus terreus

Rickettsial Arthritis

Rocky Mountain spotted fever *(Rickettsia rickettsii)*
Ehrlichia canis
Anaplasma phagocytophilium

Protozoal Arthritis

Leishmaniasis (*Leishmania* spp.)
Toxoplasmosis (rare)
Neosporosis *(Neospora caninum):* polyarthritis,
polymyositis, neurologic disease
Hepatozoonosis: polyarthritis and polymyositis in dog
and cat
Babesiosis (rare, more often causes severe anemia)

Viral Arthritis

Calicivirus infection in cats

Differential Diagnosis of Noninfectious Arthritis

Nonerosive

Immune-mediated polyarthritis
Systemic lupus erythematosus
Reactive polyarthritis (bacterial, fungal, parasitic,
neoplastic, enterohepatic, drug reaction, vaccine
induced)
Breed-associated syndromes
Polyarthritis (Akita, Newfoundland, Weimaraner)
Polyarthritis/meningitis (Akita, Beagle, Bernese
Mountain Dog, Boxer, German Shorthair Pointer)
Polyarthritis/polymyositis (spaniels)
Familial Shar-Pei fever
Lymphoplasmacytic synovitis

Erosive

Rheumatoid-like arthritis
Erosive polyarthritis of Greyhounds
Feline chronic progressive polyarthritis

Bone Disorders

Differential Diagnosis: Congenital, Developmental, Genetic

Congenital

Hemimelia, phocomelia, amelia: absence of portions or
entire limb (amelia)
Syndactyly: fusion of two or more digits; rarely clinically
significant

Polydactyly: extra digits
Ectrodactyly: third metacarpal and digit missing forming
   a cleft (split or "lobster" claw)
Segmented hemiatrophy: limb hypoplasia

Developmental and Genetic

Osteopetrosis: rare; diaphysis remains filled with bone,
   marrow does not form, fragile bones
Osteogenesis imperfecta: heritable diseases—fragile bones
Mucopolysaccharidosis: rare lysosomal storage disease—
   Siamese cats—causes dwarfism, facial dysmorphism
Dwarfism
- Osteochondrodysplasias
- Pituitary dwarfism
- Congenital hypothyroidism
Retained cartilage cores
Craniomandibular osteopathy (West Highland White
   Terrier, Scottish Terrier, Cairn Terrier, Boston Terrier,
   other terriers)
Multiple cartilaginous exostoses

Differential Diagnosis: Metabolic, Nutritional, Endocrine, Idiopathic

Metabolic

Nutritional secondary hyperparathyroidism
Lead poisoning

Nutritional

Rickets (hypovitaminosis D)
Renal osteodystrophy
Hypervitaminosis A: causes osteopathy
Hypovitaminosis A: deformed bones secondary to
   impedance of bone remodeling
Hypervitaminosis D: skeletal demineralization
Zinc-responsive chondrodysplasia
Copper deficiency
Overnutrition of growing dogs

Endocrine

Primary hyperparathyroidism
Humoral hypercalcemia of malignancy
Hyperadrenocorticism
Hypogonadism: delay in physis closure after early
   gonadectomy
Hepatic osteodystrophy
Anticonvulsant osteodystrophy

Idiopathic

Enostosis (panosteitis)

Metaphyseal osteopathy (hypertrophic osteodystrophy)

Avascular necrosis of femoral head (Legg-Calvé-Perthes disease)

Secondary hypertrophic osteopathy (usually in response to thoracic neoplasia)

Medullary bone infarction

Bone cyst

Aneurysmal bone cyst

Subchondral bone cyst

Fibrous dysplasia

Central giant cell granuloma

Liver and Exocrine Pancreatic Disorders

Cholangitis and Cholangiohepatitis, Feline

Comparative Clinical Findings

Suppurative (Neutrophilic) Cholangitis and Cholangiohepatitis

Middle-aged to older cats
Often depressed and ill
Anorexia (usually)
Jaundice
Neutrophilia
Increased alanine aminotransferase (ALT)
Increased alkaline phosphatase (ALP)
Increased bilirubin (±)
Increased serum and urine bile acids (±)
Hyperechoic liver and bile stasis
Primarily neutrophilic infiltrate
Lesions surround bile ducts
May be associated with pancreatitis and/or inflammatory bowel disease
Respond to antibiotics and supportive nonspecific treatments

Lymphocytic Cholangitis

Younger cats
Persians
Bright and alert
Polyphagia (±)

Ascites (±)
Icterus (±)
Lymphadenopathy (±)
Hepatomegaly (±)
Neutrophilia (±)
Lymphopenia (±)
Bile acids (±)
Increased ALT
Increased ALP
Bilirubinemia/bilirubinuria (±)
Hyperglobulinemia
Hyperechoic liver (±)
Primarily lymphocytic infiltrate
Lesions found in portal areas
Variable fibrosis
Pancreatitis (may be present)
Positive response to immunosuppressive corticosteroids

Exocrine Pancreatic Disease

Differential Diagnosis

Pancreatitis
- Acute
- Chronic

Exocrine pancreatic insufficiency
Pancreatic pseudocyst
Pancreatic abscess
Exocrine pancreatic neoplasia
- Pancreatic adenoma
- Pancreatic adenocarcinoma
- Pancreatic sarcoma (spindle cell sarcoma, lymphosarcoma) rare

Nodular hyperplasia
Pancreatic parasites (cats)
- *Eurytrema procyonis* (pancreatic fluke)
- *Amphimerus pseudofelineus* (hepatic fluke)

Pancreatic bladder
- Abnormal extension of pancreatic duct (rare finding in cat)

Clinical Findings of Exocrine Pancreatic Insufficiency

Most often seen in young to middle-aged dogs; German Shepherds are predisposed
Chronic weight loss

Ravenous appetite
Coprophagia
Pica
Change in fecal character
- Voluminous
- Soft
- Watery
- May be normal

Poor haircoat quality
Borborygmus, flatulence
Coagulation disorder (caused by malabsorption of vitamin
  K, rare)

Gallbladder and Extrahepatic Biliary Disease

Differential Diagnosis

Obstructive Disease
Extrahepatic biliary obstruction
- Pancreatitis (most common etiology in dog)
- Biliary neoplasia
- Cholangitis
- Pancreatic neoplasia

Cholelithiasis/choledocholithiasis
Gallbladder mucocele

Nonobstructive Disease
Cholecystitis
- Bacterial cholecystitis (ascending infection—
  Escherichia coli most common)
- Necrotizing cholecystitis
- Emphysematous cholecystitis (*E. coli, Clostridium
  perfringens*)

Cholelithiasis/choledocholithiasis (does not always cause
  obstruction)
Parasites (mainly seen in cats) Tropical climates (seen
  in cats that eat lizards or toads)
- *Platynosomum fastosum* (a fluke)
- *Amphimerus pseudofelineus*
- *Metorchis conjunctus*
- *Eurytrema procyonis*

Gallbladder infarct

Neoplasia
Biliary cystadenoma
Bile duct carcinoma

Caroli Disease
Dilatation of intrahepatic and extrahepatic bile ducts

Gallbladder Rupture
Necrotizing cholecystitis
Obstruction
Iatrogenic
Blunt abdominal trauma
Gallbladder torsion

Clinical Findings of Gallbladder and Biliary Disease

Clinical Signs
Vomiting
Icterus
Anorexia
Fever
Abdominal pain
Depression
Weight loss
Ascites/bile peritonitis

Clinicopathologic Findings
Hyperbilirubinemia
Elevated alkaline phosphatase (ALP) levels
Elevated gamma glutamyltransferase (GGT) levels
Elevated serum bile acids
Elevated alanine aminotransferase (ALT) levels
Hypercholesterolemia
Stress leukogram
Nonregenerative anemia

Radiographic Findings
Hepatomegaly
Mass effect in area of gallbladder
Gas shadow in area of gallbladder
Choleliths radiopaque if they contain calcium (50% may not be seen on radiographs)

Ultrasonographic Signs
Dilated and tortuous bile ducts
Gallbladder distension
Thickened gallbladder wall
Cholelith visible
Pancreatic mass identified
Stellate appearance to contents of gallbladder (characteristic of a gallbladder mucocele)

Hepatic Encephalopathy

Clinical Findings

General Systemic Clinical Signs
Anorexia
Depression
Weight loss
Lethargy
Nausea
Fever
Ptyalism
Intermittent vomiting
Diarrhea

Central Nervous System Clinical Signs
Tremors
Ataxia
Personality change (often toward aggression)
Dementia
Head pressing
Pacing
Circling
Hysteria
Cortical blindness
Seizures
Coma

Hepatic Lipidosis, Feline

Clinical Findings

Historical Findings
Obesity
Recent anorexia and rapid weight loss
- Concurrent disease that causes anorexia (pancreatitis, diabetes mellitus, inflammatory hepatobiliary disease, inflammatory bowel disease, feline infectious peritonitis, chronic renal failure, neoplasia, cardiomyopathy, neurologic disease, etc.)
- Stressful event
- Abrupt diet change
Typically indoor cats

Physical Findings
Jaundice
Vomiting
Dehydration

Hepatic encephalopathy
- Depression
- Ptyalism

Hepatomegaly

Clinicopathologic Findings

Typical findings of cholestasis
- Moderate increase in alanine aminotransferase (ALT)
- Marked increase in alkaline phosphatase (ALP)
- Mild increase in gamma glutamyltransferase (GGT); disproportionately low compared with other feline cholestatic hepatopathies
- Elevated serum bile acids typical

Coagulation test abnormalities (especially in conjunction with acute pancreatitis)

Cytology (Ultrasound-Guided Needle Aspirates) and Histopathology

Reveal clear vacuolation of most hepatocytes, nonzonal in distribution; typically with absence of inflammatory cells

Hepatobiliary Disease

Clinical and Physical Findings

General Clinical Features

Depression
Anorexia
Lethargy
Weight loss
Poor haircoat, insufficient grooming
Nausea, vomiting
Diarrhea
Dehydration
Small body stature
Polydipsia, polyuria

Signs Specific but Not Pathognomonic for Hepatic Disease

Icterus
Bilirubinuria
Acholic feces
Organomegaly
Ascites
Hepatic encephalopathy
- Behavioral changes (aggression, dementia, hysteria)
- Circling
- Ataxia

- Staggering
- Pacing
- Head pressing
- Cortical blindness
- Ptyalism
- Tremors/seizures
- Coma

Coagulopathies

Polydipsia/polyuria

Causes of Elevated Serum Hepatobiliary Enzymes

Primary Hepatic Disease

Drug Induction

Corticosteroids (dogs)

Anticonvulsants (phenobarbital, phenytoin, primidone)

Endocrinopathies

Hyperadrenocorticism (dogs)

Hypothyroidism (dogs)

Hyperthyroidism (cats)

Diabetes mellitus

Bone Disorders

Growing animals

Osteosarcoma

Osteomyelitis

Neoplasia

Adenocarcinomas (pancreatic, intestinal, adrenocortical, mammary)

Sarcomas (hemangiosarcoma, leiomyosarcoma)

Hepatic metastasis

Muscle Injury

Acute muscle necrosis/trauma

Myopathies

Malignant hyperthermia

Hypoxia/Hypotension

Septic shock

Surgery

Congestive heart failure

Hypoadrenocorticism

Circulatory shock

Severe acute blood loss

Hypotensive crisis

Status epilepticus

Gastrointestinal Disease
Pancreatitis
Inflammatory bowel disease

Miscellaneous Causes
Systemic infections
Pregnancy (cats—increased placental alkaline phosphatase)
Colostrum-fed neonates (dogs)
Breed related (Scottish terrier)

Differential Diagnosis, Dogs

Inflammation
Chronic hepatitis complex
- Copper accumulation—Bedlington Terrier, Airedale Terrier, Bull Terrier, Bulldog, Cocker Spaniel, Collie, Dachshund, Dalmatian, Doberman Pinscher, German Shepherd, Golden Retriever, Keeshond, Kerry Blue Terrier, Labrador Retriever, Norwich Terrier, Old English Sheepdog, Pekingese, Poodle, Samoyed, Schnauzer, Skye Terrier, West Highland White Terrier, Wire Fox Terrier
- Drug induced: trimethoprim-sulfa, phenobarbital, diethylcarbamazine, oxibendazole, many others
- Familial hepatitis—Doberman Pinscher, West Highland White Terrier, Dalmatian, Skye Terrier, Cocker Spaniel

Fibrosis and cirrhosis (results from any severe or chronic hepatic insult)
Infectious agents: leptospirosis, canine adenovirus type 1 infection, bacterial hepatitis, histoplasmosis, Rocky Mountain spotted fever, ehrlichiosis, babesiosis, leishmaniasis
Cholangiohepatitis
Granulomatous hepatitis
- *Rhodococcus, Borrelia, Bartonella, Histoplasma, Coccidioidomyces, Hepatozoon, Heterobilharzia Nocardia, Mycobacterium* spp.

Acidophil cell hepatitis
Lobular dissecting hepatitis
Hepatic abscess

Acute Toxic or Drug-Induced Hepatopathy

Vacuolar Hepatopathy

Metabolic Liver Disease
Amyloidosis
Hyperlipidemia
Lysosomal storage disease

Vascular Hepatic Disease
   Congenital portosystemic venous anomaly
   Intrahepatic portal vein hypoplasia
   Intrahepatic arteriovenous fistula

Biliary Tract Disease

Neoplasia
   Primary: hepatocellular carcinoma, hepatocellular
      adenoma, hepatic hemangiosarcoma, biliary carcinoma
   Other hepatic tumors: leiomyosarcoma, liposarcoma, myxo-
      sarcoma, fibrosarcoma, biliary adenoma, hepatic carcinoid
   Hemolymphatic: lymphosarcoma, mast cell tumor,
      plasma cell tumor
   Metastatic neoplasia

Hepatic or Biliary Cysts

Differential Diagnosis, Cats

Hepatic Lipidosis

Inflammatory Hepatobiliary Disease
   Cholangitis/cholangiohepatitis complex
   • Suppurative (neutrophilic) cholangitis,
      cholangiohepatitis
   • Lymphocytic cholangitis
   Chronic cholangiohepatitis (later stage of acute
      cholangiohepatitis)
   Sclerosing cholangitis
   Lymphocytic portal hepatitis
   Feline infectious peritonitis (FIP)

Toxic Hepatopathy
   Antimicrobials (trimethoprim-sulfa, tetracycline)
   Anticonvulsants (phenobarbital)
   Diazepam
   Methimazole
   Griseofulvin
   Ketoconazole
   Pine oils (cleaning agents)
   Amanita phalloides (death cap mushroom)
   Natural or herbal remedies
   Many others

Portosystemic Venous Anomaly

Lipoprotein Lipase Deficiency

Neoplasia
   Primary Hepatic Neoplasia
      Biliary carcinoma
      Hepatocellular carcinoma

Hepatic hemangiosarcoma
Bilary cystadenoma
Myelolipoma
Hepatic carcinoid

Hemolymphatic Neoplasia
Lymphosarcoma
Mast cell tumor
Plasma cell tumor

Metastatic Neoplasia

Hepatomegaly and Microhepatica

Differential Diagnosis

Generalized Hepatomegaly
Acute toxic hepatopathy
Infiltrative hepatic disease
- Neoplasia: primary or metastatic
- Chronic hepatitis complex (dog)
- Cholangiohepatitis (cat)
- Extramedullary hematopoiesis
- Mononuclear-phagocytic cell hyperplasia
- Amyloidosis (rare)
Passive congestion
- Right-sided heart failure
- Pericardial disease (dog)
- Caval syndrome (dog)
- Caudal vena cava obstruction (dog)
- Budd-Chiari syndrome (rare)
Hepatocellular hypertrophy
- Hepatic lipidosis
- Steroid hepatopathy
- Anticonvulsant drug therapy
Acute extrahepatic bile duct obstruction

Focal Hepatomegaly
Neoplasia: primary or metastatic
Nodular hyperplasia
Chronic hepatic disease with fibrosis and nodular regeneration
Hepatic abscess
Hepatic cyst

Microhepatica
Decreased hepatic mass
- Chronic hepatic disease with progressive loss of hepatocytes

Decreased portal blood flow with hepatocellular atrophy
- Congenital portosystemic shunt
- Intrahepatic portal vein hypoplasia
- Chronic portal vein thrombosis

Hypovolemia
- Hypoadrenocorticism
- Shock

Hyperlipidemia

Differential Diagnosis

Postprandial Hyperlipidemia

Primary

Idiopathic hyperlipoproteinemia of Miniature Schnauzers
Feline familial hyperchylomicronemia
Idiopathic hypercholesterolemia (rare—Doberman Pinscher, Rottweiler)
Idiopathic hypercholesterolemia

Secondary

Endocrine
- Hypothyroidism
- Diabetes mellitus
- Hyperadrenocorticism

Pancreatitis
Nephrotic syndrome
Hepatic insufficiency
Cholestasis
Drug induced
- Glucocorticoids
- Megesterol acetate

Clinical Findings

Severe Hyperlipidemia

Intermittent gastrointestinal signs
- Vomiting
- Diarrhea
- Abdominal discomfort

Seizures
Pancreatitis
Lipemia retinalis
Cutaneous xanthomas
Peripheral nerve paralysis
Behavioral changes

Severe Hypercholesterolemia
>   Arcus lipoides corneae
>   Lipemia retinalis
>   Atherosclerosis

Pancreatitis

Clinical Findings of Acute Pancreatitis

Dogs

Mild Acute Pancreatitis

>   Depression
>   Anorexia
>   Nausea, vomiting, diarrhea
>   Ptyalism
>   Mild right cranial abdominal pain
>   Fever, dehydration, weakness

Moderate to Severe Acute Pancreatitis

>   Depression
>   Anorexia
>   Vomiting
>   Right cranial abdominal pain
>   Hematemesis, hematochezia, melena
>   Jaundice
>   Respiratory distress
>   Shock, fever, dehydration
>   Hyperemic mucous membranes
>   Tachycardia, tachypnea
>   Abdominal effusion
>   Mass effect in region of pancreas
>   Petechiae, ecchymoses
>   Cardiac arrhythmia
>   Glossitis, glossal slough
>   Extrahepatic biliary obstruction

Cats

>   Signs tend to be more subclinical and nonspecific.
>   May be associated with inflammatory bowel disease
>   May be component of multisystemic disease such as toxoplasmosis
>   Lethargy, anorexia, vomiting, dehydration, weight loss, jaundice, hypothermia
>   May present as acute necrotizing or acute suppurative form

Predisposing Factors

Nutritional
Obesity
High-fat diet
After ingestion of large, fatty meal

Hypertriglyceridemia
Hyperlipoproteinemia (Idiopathic in Miniature Schnauzers)
Endocrine (diabetes mellitus, hyperadrenocorticism, hypothyroidism)

Drugs
Chemotherapeutic agents
- L-Asparaginase
- Azathioprine
- Others

Organophosphates
Asparaginase
Thiazides
Furosemide
Estrogens
Sulfa drugs
Procainamide
Potassium bromide
Tetracyclines

Ischemia
Hypovolemia
Associated with disseminated intravascular coagulation (DIC)
Vasoactive amine–induced vasoconstriction
Surgery
Gastric dilatation/volvulus
Severe immune-mediated hemolytic anemia

Duodenal Reflex
Increased intraluminal pressure during severe vomiting

Other
Cholangitis
Infection (toxoplasmosis, feline infectious peritonitis)
Abdominal trauma
Hypercalcemia
Trauma

Clinicopathologic Findings in Dogs and Cats with Acute Pancreatitis

- BUN/creatinine—increased in 50 to 65% of dogs and in 33% (Cr) and 57% (BUN) in cats. Usually prerenal due to dehydration and hypotension. May be secondary to intrinsic renal failure (sepsis and immune-complex)
- Potassium—decreased in 20% of cases in dogs and 56% in cats. Increased loss in vomiting and due to renal loss with fluid therapy plus reduced intake and aldosterone release caused by hypovolemia
- Sodium—can be increased, decreased or normal. Increase usually caused by dehydration, decrease caused by losses secondary to vomiting
- Calcium—Commonly decreased in cats, rarely in dogs, rarely increased in both dogs and cats. Reduction is a poor prognostic indicator in cats but no prognostic significance in dogs. May be caused by saponification in peripancreatic fat and glucagon release stimulating calcitonin
- Chloride—Very commonly decreased in dogs. Loss in gastrointestinal secretions in vomiting
- Phosphate—Often increased in dogs, uncommonly increased or decreased in cats. Increase usually due to reduced renal excretion secondary to renal compromise. Decrease (in cats) due to treatment for diabetes mellitus
- Glucose—increased in 40-88% of dogs and decreased in up to 40%. Increased in 64% of cats, rarely decreased. Increase due to decreased insulin and increased glucagon, cortisol, and catecholamines. Decrease caused by sepsis or anorexia
- Albumin—Increased in 39-50% and decreased in 17% of dogs. Increased in 8-30% and decreased in 40% of cats. Increase due to dehydration. Decrease due to gut loss, malnutrition, concurrent hepatic disease, or renal loss
- Hepatocellular enzymes (ALT, AST)—increased in 61% of dogs and 68% of cats. Hepatic necrosis and vacuolation due to sepsis, local effects of pancreatitis +/- concurrent hepatic disease in cats
- Cholestatic enzymes (ALP and GGT)—Increased in 79% of dogs and 50% of cats. Biliary obstruction due to acute or chronic pancreatitis +/- concurrent cholangitis +/- lipidosis in cats; steroid-induced ALP in dogs
- Bilirubin—Increased in 53% of dogs and 64% of cats (same causes as GGT and ALP)

- Cholesterol—Increased in 48-80% of dogs and 64% of cats. Can be due to cholestasis; unclear if cause or effect
- Triglycerides—Commonly increased in dogs. Unclear if cause or effect
- Neutrophils—Increased in 55-60% of dogs, increased in 30% and decreased in 15% of cats. Increased due to inflammatory response. Decreased in some cats due to consumption, may be a poor prognostic indicator
- Hematocrit—Increased in about 20% and decreased in 20% of both dogs and cats. Increased due to dehydration and decreased due to anemia of chronic disease or gastric ulceration
- Platelets—Commonly decreased in severe cases in dogs. Decreased due to circulating proteases +/− disseminated intravascular coagulation

Portosystemic Shunt, Congenital

Clinical Findings

Signalment
Young animal, male or female, often purebred

History
Neurologic signs (dementia, circling, central blindness, personality change, head pressing, wall hugging, seizures)
Vomiting
Diarrhea
Ptyalism (especially cats)
Worsening of signs after eating
Improvement of signs with antimicrobial therapy
Prolonged recovery from anesthesia
Polydipsia/polyuria
Recurrent urate urolithiasis in breeds other than Dalmatian and English Bulldog

Physical Examination
Poor haircoat
Small stature
Cystic calculi
Cryptorchidism
Bilateral renomegaly
Copper-colored irises in non-Asian cat breeds
Other congenital anomalies

Clinicopathologic Findings
Microcytosis
Hypoalbuminemia
Mild increases in hepatic enzymes
Hypocholesterolemia
Low BUN
Normal to high resting bile acids/elevated postprandial bile acids
Hyposthenuria
Urate crystalluria and urolithiasis

Vacuolar Hepatopathy, Canine

Differential Diagnosis

Hyperadrenocorticism
- Pituitary dependent
- Adrenal dependent
- Iatrogenic (glucocorticoid therapy)

Pancreatitis
- Chronic

Severe hypothyroidism

Chronic stress
- Illness of more than 4 months

Chronic infection or inflammation (e.g., pyelonephritis, chronic dermatitis)

Severe dental disease
- Oral infection

Disorders affecting lipid metabolism
- Diabetes mellitus
- Idiopathic hyperlipidemia

Neoplasia
- Lymphoma

Congestive heart failure

Abnormal sex hormone production

Inflammatory bowel disease
- Chronic, lymphoplasmacytic, eosinophilic

Hepatocutaneous syndrome

Neoplasia

Chemotherapeutic Agent Toxicity

Most severely affects tissues with a growth fraction that approaches that of tumor cells

Clinical Findings

Myelosuppression

Neutropenia: short-lived cells; nadir is 5-10 days postchemotherapy

Thrombocytopenia: nadir is 7-14 days postchemotherapy

Anemia: erythrocytes live longer; rarely clinically significant

Gastrointestinal Toxicity

Nausea, vomiting

Diarrhea

Inappetence

Anorexia

Cardiotoxicity

Doxorubicin therapy

Breeds susceptible to dilated cardiomyopathy (e.g., Doberman) most sensitive

Most likely after cumulative dose of 180 mg/m^2

Nephrotoxicity

Cisplatin, streptozotocin

Limit use of cisplatin in cases of preexisting renal disease.

Hepatopathy

Irreversible hepatic toxicity may result if lomustine (CCNU) given in face of elevated ALT

Urothelial Toxicity

Sterile hemorrhagic cystitis
Cyclophosphamide, ifosfamide

Extravasation

Doxorubicin: severe local reaction leading to slough
Vincristine: usually minor tissue damage

Hypersensitivity

Doxorubicin: caused by histamine release from mast cells;
prevented by slow administration

L-Asparaginase: less likely if given subcutaneously rather
than intravenously

Etoposide, paclitaxel: caused by carrier solutions for these
agents

Alopecia

Less of a problem in dogs and cats than in people
Worse in breeds that have hair (e.g., Poodles, Terriers, Old
English Sheepdogs) than in dogs with fur
Loss of "feathers" (e.g., Golden Retrievers)
Loss of whiskers in cats

Neurologic Toxicity

Fatal neurotoxicity in cats with topical or systemic
administration of 5-fluorouracil

Respiratory Toxicity

Fatal, acute pulmonary edema in cats with cisplatin therapy

Corticosteroid Therapy

Adverse Effects Associated with Glucocorticoid Administration

Polyuria/polydipsia
Polyphagia
Increased alkaline phosphatase (ALP) levels
Increased gamma glutamyltransferase (GGT) levels
Panting
Insomnia, agitation, behavioral changes
Immunosuppression
- Secondary infection
- Recrudescence of latent infection
- Worsening of existing infection
- Demodicosis
Vacuolar hepatopathy
Iatrogenic hyperadrenocorticism
Adrenocorticoid deficiency with rapid withdrawal after
sustained use

Alopecia
Calcinosis cutis
Comedones
Skin thinning
Proteinuria
Muscle atrophy/muscle wasting
Myotonia/myopathy
Delayed wound healing
Colonic perforation
Gastrointestinal ulceration
Insulin resistance
Diabetes mellitus
Hyperlipidemia
Abortion
Growth suppression
Hypercoagulable state
Ligament and tendon rupture
Psychosis/behavior change
Lowered seizure threshold
Osteopenia

Histiocytic Disease

Classification, Dogs

May be difficult to differentiate from lymphoproliferative, granulo-matous, or reactive inflammatory disease by histopathology alone

Cutaneous Histiocytoma
>Benign, usually solitary lesion
>Typically young dogs
>Often spontaneously regress

Langerhans Cell Histiocytoma
>Rare, rapidly metastatic, cutaneous infiltration by
>histiocytes, may be limited to multiple cutaneous sites
>or may affect lymph nodes and internal organs

Cutaneous Histiocytosis
>Single or multiple lesions
>May spontaneously regress
>May respond to immunosuppressive drugs

Systemic Histiocytosis
>Familial disease of Bernese Mountain Dogs, rarely other breeds
>Similar lesions to cutaneous histiocytosis but may also
>affect mucous membranes, lymphoid organs, lung,
>bone marrow, and other organ systems
>Progressive, requires immunosuppressive therapy

Histiocytic Sarcoma

Bernese Mountain Dog, Rottweiler, Flat-Coated Retriever, Golden Retriever, rarely other breeds

Histiocytic sarcoma usually begins as a localized lesion in spleen, lymph nodes, lung, bone marrow, skin and subcutis, brain, and periarticular tissue of appendicular joints.

- Rapidly disseminates to multiple organs

Malignant Histiocytosis

Bernese Mountain Dog, Rottweiler, Flat-Coated Retriever, Golden Retriever, rarely other breeds

Multisystemic, rapidly progressive disease of multiple organs

Classification, Cats

Feline Progressive Histiocytosis

Rare, usually see multiple skin nodules, papules, plaques

Head, lower extremities, trunk

Poor long-term prognosis

Feline Histiocytic Sarcoma

Poorly demarcated tumors of subcutis or spleen

Poor prognosis

Humoral Hypercalcemia

Differential Diagnosis

Hematologic Cancers

- Lymphosarcoma
- Lymphocytic leukemia
- Myeloproliferative disease
- Myeloma

Solid Tumors with Bone Metastasis

- Mammary adenocarcinoma
- Nasal adenocarcinoma
- Epithelial-derived tumors
- Pancreatic adenocarcinoma
- Lung carcinoma

Solid Tumors without Bone Metastasis

- Apocrine gland adenocarcinoma of the anal sac
- Interstitial cell tumor
- Squamous cell carcinoma
- Thyroid adenocarcinoma

- Lung carcinoma
- Pancreatic adenocarcinoma
- Fibrosarcoma

Lymphoma

Common Differential Diagnoses

Generalized Lymphadenopathy
Disseminated infections
- Bacterial, fungal, rickettsial, parasitic, viral

Immune-mediated disease
- Systemic lupus erythematosus (SLE), polyarthritis vasculitis, dermatopathy

Other hematopoietic tumors
- Leukemia, multiple myeloma, malignant or systemic histiocytosis

Neoplasia metastatic to lymph nodes
Benign reactive hyperplastic syndromes in cats

Alimentary Disease
Inflammatory bowel diseases
- Lymphocytic/plasmacytic, eosinophilic enteritis

Nonlymphoid intestinal neoplasia
Granulomatous enteritis
Granulated round cell tumors in cats
Gastrointestinal mast cell neoplasia in cats

Cutaneous Disease
Infectious dermatitis (deep pyoderma, fungal dermatitis)
Immune-mediated dermatitis (e.g., pemphigus foliaceus)
Other cutaneous neoplasms

Mediastinal Disease
Thymoma
Chemodectoma (heart base tumor)
Ectopic thyroid neoplasia
Pulmonary lymphomatoid granulomatosis
Granulomatous disease (e.g., hilar lymphadenopathy with blastomycosis)

Paraneoplastic Syndromes

Classification

General
Cancer anorexia, cachexia
Fever

Hematologic

Anemia
- Anemia of chronic disease
- Immune-mediated hemolytic anemia
- Bone marrow infiltration
- Blood loss anemia
- Hyperestrogenism
- Microangiopathic hemolytic anemia

Polycythemia (rare)
- Associated with renal neoplasia, nasal fibrosarcoma, lymphoma, bronchial carcinoma, cecal leiomyosarcoma, transmissible venereal tumor, schwannoma

Leukocytosis
- Neutrophilic
- Eosinophilic

Thrombocytopenia
- Increased consumption
- Decreased production (bone marrow neoplasia)
- Increased destruction (immune-mediated thrombocytopenia)

Thrombocytosis

Thrombocyte hyperaggregability/hypercoagulability

Pancytopenia

Coagulation disorders
- Disseminated intravascular coagulation (DIC)
- Coagulation-activating substances produced by tumor

Hyperproteinemia/hyperglobulinemia

Endocrine

Hypercalcemia of malignancy

Hypoglycemia

Syndrome of inappropriate antidiuretic hormone (ADH) secretion
- Hyponatremia, serum
- Hypoosmolality, urine
- Hyperosmolality

Hyperestrogenism (Sertoli cell tumor)

Gastrointestinal

Gastroduodenal ulceration
- Mast cell tumors, gastrinoma

Cancer cachexia

Renal

Glomerulonephritis

Hypercalcemic nephropathy

Cutaneous
   Superficial necrolytic dermatitis
   Nodular dermatofibrosis
   Feline paraneoplastic alopecia

Neuromuscular
   Myasthenia gravis
   • Dogs with thymoma
   Peripheral neuropathy
   • Multiple myeloma, lymphoma, various carcinomas and sarcomas

Hypertrophic Osteodystrophy
   Space-occupying mass in thorax or rarely abdomen

Sarcomas

Classification of Soft Tissue Sarcomas

Fibrosarcoma
Mast cell tumor
Undifferentiated sarcoma
Hemangiosarcoma
Hemangiopericytoma (peripheral nerve-sheath tumor)
Myxosarcoma
Leiomyosarcoma
Malignant fibrous histiocytoma
Schwannoma
Neurofibrosarcoma
Synovial cell sarcoma
Rhabdomyosarcoma
Liposarcoma
Vaccine-associated fibrosarcoma (cats)

Clinical Findings for Hemangiosarcoma

Older dogs and cats
Many potential sites of origin
• Spleen
• Right atrium
• Subcutis
• Pericardium
• Liver
• Muscle
• Lung
• Skin
• Bone
• Kidney
• Central nervous system

- Peritoneum
- Oral cavity
- Nasal cavity
- Eye
- Retroperitoneum

Hemoabdomen
Pericardial effusion
Cardiac tamponade
Sudden death
Anorexia, vomiting
Lethargy
Right-sided heart failure
Muffled heart sounds
Arrhythmias
Neurologic signs (may metastasize to brain)

Thyroid Neoplasms

Classification and Clinical Findings

Cats

Hyperthyroidism: functional thyroid tumors
- Thyroid adenoma
- Thyroid adenocarcinoma

Dogs

Nonfunctional Tumors (90%)

Thyroid adenoma
Thyroid adenocarcinoma
- Swelling or mass in neck
- Dyspnea
- Cough
- Lethargy
- Dysphagia
- Regurgitation
- Anorexia
- Weight loss
- Horner syndrome
- Change in bark
- Facial edema

Functional Tumors (10%)

Thyroid adenoma
Thyroid adenocarcinoma
- Swelling or mass in neck
- Polyphagia/weight
- Hyperactivity

- Polyuria/polydipsia
- Panting
- Change in behavior (aggression)

Tumors

Bone and Joint Tumors, Classification

Canine osteosarcoma
    Appendicular
    Skull
    Scapular
    Pelvic
    Ribs
    Vertebral
    Nasal and paranasal
Chondrosarcoma
Fibrosarcoma
Hemangiosarcoma
Multilobular osteochondrosarcoma
Osteoma
Canine multiple cartilaginous exostoses
Feline osteosarcoma
Feline multiple cartilaginous exostoses
Metastatic bone tumors
    Transitional cell carcinoma
    Prostatic adenocarcinoma
    Mammary carcinoma
    Thyroid carcinoma
    Pulmonary carcinoma
    Nasal carcinoma
    Apocrine gland, anal sac adenocarcinoma
    Renal tumors
    Others
Primary joint tumors
    Synovial cell sarcoma
    Histiocytic sarcoma
    Malignant fibrous histiocytoma
    Synovial myxoma
    Myxosarcoma
    Osteosarcoma
    Fibrosarcoma
    Chondrosarcoma
    Hemangiosarcoma
    Liposarcoma
    Rhabdomyosarcoma
    Undifferentiated sarcoma

Hematopoietic Tumors, Classification

Lymphoma

Feline

Alimentary

Multicentric

Mediastinal/thymic

Nasal

Renal

Other

Feline leukemia virus (FeLV) associated

Canine

Multicentric

Others (alimentary, mediastinal, cutaneous)

Lymphoid Leukemia

Acute lymphoblastic leukemia (in cats, often associated with FeLV infection)

Chronic lymphocytic leukemia

Nonlymphoid Leukemias and Myeloproliferative Disorders

Acute myelogenous leukemia (myeloblastic)

Acute myelomonocytic leukemia (myeloblasts/ monoblasts)

Acute monocytic leukemia (monoblasts)

Acute megakaryoblastic leukemia (megakaryoblasts)

Erythroleukemia (erythroblasts)

Chronic Myeloproliferative Disorders

Chronic myelogenous leukemia (neutrophils, late precursors)

Primary thrombocythemia (platelets)

Basophilic leukemia (basophils and precursors)

Eosinophic leukemia (eosinophils and precursors)

Polycythemia vera (erythrocytes)

Plasma Cell Neoplasms

Multiple myeloma

Solitary plasmacytoma

IgM (Waldenström macroglobulinemia)

Mast Cell Tumor (MCT) Disease, Clinical Findings

Clinical Appearance and Location of MCTs

Extremely variable in appearance

Soft, fluctuant, firm, discrete, diffuse, small, large, solitary, multiple, haired, hairless, dermal, or subcutaneous

Erythema, bruising, ulceration

On trunk most often; also perineum, extremities, head, neck

Rarely oral cavity, nasal cavity, larynx, conjunctiva

Systemic Signs of Disseminated Mastocytosis

Gastrointestinal ulceration
Abdominal discomfort
Vomiting
Melena
Hypotension
Coagulation abnormalities
Acute or chronic blood loss anemia

Oral Cavity Tumors, Differential Diagnosis

Malignant Neoplasms

Melanoma
Squamous cell carcinoma
Fibrosarcoma
Osteosarcoma
Lingual carcinoma or sarcoma
Histiocytic sarcoma
Lymphoma
Mast cell tumor

Benign Neoplasms

Epulides (acanthomatous ameloblastoma)
- Fibromatous
- Ossifying
- Acanthomatous (squamous): may be invasive but does not metastasize

Papillomas: self-limiting
Fibroma
Lipoma
Chondroma
Osteoma
Odontoma
Cementoma
Plasmacytoma
Hemangioma
Hemangiopericytoma
Histiocytoma
Eosinophilic granuloma

Skin and Subcutaneous Tumors

Epithelial Tumors

Sebaceous gland adenoma/adenocarcinoma
Squamous cell carcinoma

- Canine cutaneous squamous cell carcinoma
- Canine nasal planum squamous cell carcinoma
- Canine digital squamous cell carcinoma
- Feline cutaneous squamous cell carcinoma
- Feline multicentric squamous cell carcinoma in situ (Bowen disease)

Trichoepithelioma
Intracutaneous cornifying epithelioma
Basal cell tumors
- Benign tumors
- Basal carcinoma

Trichoblastoma
Pilomatricoma
Papilloma
Perianal gland tumors (hepatoid gland tumors)
Sweat gland tumors (apocrine gland tumors)
Ceruminous gland tumors
Anal sac, apocrine gland tumors
Follicular stem cell carcinoma

Round Cell Tumors

Lymphoma
Mast cell tumor
Histiocytoma
Transmissible venereal tumor (TVT)
Plasmacytoma

Melanocytic Tumors

Melanoma
- Benign (typically melanomas of haired skin and eyelids)
- Malignant (typically those of digit or mucocutaneous junctions)

Urogenital Tumors, Classification

Kidney

Lymphoma (most common renal tumor in cats)
Primary renal carcinoma, adenoma/adenocarcinoma
Cystadenocarcinoma with concurrent nodular dermatofibrosis in German Shepherds
Tumors of embryonic origin (e.g., Wilm tumor)
Nephroblastoma
Transitional cell carcinoma

Urinary Bladder

Older female dogs, West Highland White Terrier, Scottish Terriers, Beagles, Dachshunds, Shetland Sheepdogs
Transitional cell carcinoma

Squamous cell carcinoma
Leiomyosarcoma
Leiomyoma
Rhabdomyosarcoma
Metastatic neoplasia
- Hemangiosarcoma
- Lymphoma
- Extension of prostate neoplasia

Prostate

Prostatic adenocarcinoma
Transitional cell carcinoma

Penis and Prepuce

Prepuce affected by tumors of haired skin seen
   elsewhere
Penile
- Transmissible venereal tumor
- Others

Testicular Neoplasia

Cryptorchid dogs are 13.6 times more likely to develop
   Sertoli cell tumor or seminoma
Sertoli cell tumor (25-50% are functional and cause
   hyperestrogenemia)
Leydig cell (interstitial) tumor
Seminoma

Vagina and Vulva

Leiomyoma
Fibroleiomyoma
Fibroma
Polyps
Lipoma
Leiomyosarcoma (rare)
Transmissible venereal tumor (TVT)

Uterus

Leiomyoma
Leiomyosarcoma
Uterine adenocarcinoma

Ovary

Epithelial Tumors (50% of ovarian tumors)
   Papillary adenoma
   Cystadenoma
   Papillary adenocarcinoma
   Undifferentiated adenocarcinoma

Germ Cell Tumors (10% of ovarian tumors)
Dysgerminoma
Teratoma
Teratocarcinoma

Sex-Cord Stromal Tumors (40% of ovarian tumors)
Granulosa cell tumor
Benign thecoma
Benign luteoma

Mammary Gland
Fibroadenoma (mixed mammary tumor)
Solid carcinomas
Tubular adenocarcinoma
Sarcoma
Inflammatory carcinomas
Feline mammary adenocarcinomas

Neurologic and Neuromuscular Disorders

Brain Disease, Congenital or Hereditary

Differential Diagnosis

Congenital Malformations

Failure of normal closure of neural tube: vary in severity from clinically inapparent (agenesis of corpus callosum) to severe (anencephaly)

Lissencephaly: failure of normal migration of neurons in development of cerebral cortex; leads to abnormal appearance of sulci and gyri (most often seen in Lhasa Apso)

Cerebellar hypoplasia: seen most often in cats after in utero panleukopenia infection; rarely seen with parvovirus infection of developing cerebellum in dogs; may be isolated malformation without infection

Chiari-like malformations: protrusion of cerebellar vermis through foramen magnum (Cavalier King Charles Spaniel, other dog breeds)

Hydrocephalus: congenital hydrocephalus seen most often in toy and brachycephalic breeds; suggests hereditary basis; often congenital stenosis or aplasia of mesencephalic aqueducts

Inborn errors of metabolism (hereditary): young, purebred animals with diffuse, symmetric signs of brain disease
- Organic acidurias
- Spongiform encephalopathies: may be hereditary or acquired (transmissible) disease
- Polioencephalopathies: metabolic defects that affect gray matter
- Neuroaxonal dystrophy: spheroids causing swelling within axons
- Leukoencephalopathies: disorders of myelin; affect white matter; often affect cerebellum and long tracts leading to tremors and dysmetria
- Lysosomal storage diseases: accumulation of metabolic products in lysosomes
- Ceroid lipofuscinosis: accumulation of proteins in lysosomes
- Neonatal encephalopathy: hereditary disease of Standard Poodles

Movement Disorders

Hereditary cerebellar hypoplasia

Multisystem degeneration: diseases of cerebellum and basal ganglia—progressive neuronal abiotrophy of Kerry Blue Terriers and Chinese Crested dogs

Dyskinesis and dystonias

Paroxysmal dyskinesias ("Scotty cramp" or idiopathic cerebellitis)—Scottish Terriers

Cognitive Dysfunction

Clinical Findings

Disorientation

Sleep/wake cycle alterations

House soiling problems

Change in activity levels
- Increased
- Stereotypic
- Decreased

Agitation

Anxiety

Altered responsiveness to stimuli
- Heightened
- Reduced

Changes in appetite
- Increased
- Decreased

Decreased ability to perform learned tasks
Changes in interaction with owners

Cranial Nerve (CN) Deficits

Clinical Findings

CN I (Olfactory)
Loss of ability to smell

CN II (Optic)
Loss of vision, loss of menace response, dilated pupil, loss of papillary light reflex (direct and consensual)

CN III (Oculomotor)
Loss of papillary light reflex on affected side (even if light shone in opposite eye), dilated pupil, ptosis, ventrolateral strabismus

CN IV (Trochlear)
Slight dorsomedial eye rotation

CN V (Trigeminal)
Atrophy of temporalis and masseter muscles, loss of jaw tone and strength, dropped jaw (if bilateral), analgesia of innervated areas

CN VI (Abducens)
Medial strabismus, impaired lateral gaze, poor retraction of globe

CN VII (Facial)
Lip, eyelid, and ear droop; loss of ability to blink; loss of ability to retract lip; possibly decreased tear production

CN VIII (Vestibulocochlear)
Ataxia, head tilt, nystagmus, deafness, positional strabismus

CN IX (Glossopharyngeal)
Loss of gag reflex, dysphagia

CN X (Vagus)
Loss of gag reflex, laryngeal paralysis, dysphagia, megaesophagus

CN XI (Accessory)
Atrophy of trapezius, sternocephalicus, and brachiocephalicus muscles

CN XII (Hypoglossal)
Loss of tongue strength, inability to retract tongue if bilateral, atrophy of tongue

Head Tilt

Differential Diagnosis

Peripheral Vestibular Disease
Otitis media/interna
Feline idiopathic vestibular disease
Geriatric canine vestibular disease
Feline nasopharyngeal polyps
Middle ear tumor
- Ceruminous gland adenocarcinoma
- Squamous cell carcinoma

Trauma
Aminoglycoside ototoxicity/chemical ototoxicity
Hypothyroidism (possibly)

Central Vestibular Disease
Trauma/hemorrhage
Infectious inflammatory disease
- Rocky Mountain spotted fever
- Feline infectious peritonitis (FIP)
- Others

Granulomatous meningoencephalitis
Neoplasia
Vascular infarct
Thiamine deficiency
Metronidazole toxicity

Inflammatory Disease of the Nervous System

Differential Diagnosis

Steroid-responsive meningitis-arteritis (steroid-responsive
suppurative meningitis) (juvenile to young adult large breed
dogs: Bernese Mountain Dogs, Boxers, German Shorthaired
Pointers, Nova Scotia Duck Tolling Retrievers)
Granulomatous meningoencephalitis
- Idiopathic inflammatory brain disease of dogs
- Most commonly in small breed dogs

Pug meningoencephalitis
- Necrotizing meningoencephalitis of cerebral cortex
- Maltese and Yorkshire terrier also

Feline polioencephalomyelitis
- Young cats, progressive course

Feline immunodeficiency virus (FIV) encephalopathy
Bacterial meningitis and myelitis
- *Staphylococcus aureus*
- *Staphylococcus epidermidis*

- *Staphylococcus albus*
- *Pasteurella multocida*
- *Actinomyces*
- *Nocardia*
- Others

Canine distemper virus

Rabies

Feline infectious peritonitis (FIP)

Toxoplasmosis

Neosporosis

Borreliosis

Mycotic infections

- *Cryptococcus neoformans, C. gattii*
- Other disseminated systemic mycoses

Rickettsial diseases

- Rocky Mountain spotted fever
- Ehrlichiosis
- *Ehrlichia ewingii, Anaplasma phagocytophilia*

Parasitic meningitis, myelitis, encephalitis

- Aberrant parasite migration

Intracranial Neoplasms

Differential Diagnosis

Meningioma
Benign tumor of cells of meninges

Neuroepithelial Tumors (Gliomas)
Astrocytomas

Oligodendrogliomas

Choroid plexus tumors (choroid plexus papilloma, ependymal tumor)

Central Nervous System (CNS) Lymphoma
Primary: neoplasia of native CNS lymphocytes

Secondary: metastasis of systemic lymphoma

Metastatic Neoplasia to CNS
Local invasion: nasal adenocarcinoma

Hematogenous spread: melanoma, hemangiosarcoma, lymphosarcoma

Many other neoplasms may metastasize to CNS.

Pituitary Tumors
Functional tumors of pars distalis or pars intermedius: cause pituitary-dependent hyperadrenocorticism; generally cause little damage to surrounding tissue

Pituitary macrotumor

Myasthenia Gravis

Congenital myasthenia gravis: inherited deficiency of acetylcholine receptors at presynaptic membranes of skeletal muscle.

Acquired myasthenia gravis: antibodies made against nicotinic acetylcholine receptors of skeletal muscle.

Clinical Findings

Appendicular muscle weakness
- Worsens with exercise
- Improves with rest
- Tetraplegia

Mentation, postural reactions, reflexes normal

Megaesophagus
- Salivation
- Regurgitation

Dysphagia

Ventroflexion

Urinary bladder distension

Hoarse bark or meow

Persistently dilated pupils

Facial muscle weakness

Aspiration pneumonia

Respiratory weakness

Myositis and Myopathies

Differential Diagnosis

Inflammatory Myopathies

Masticatory myositis
- Immunoglobulin G (IgG) antibodies to type 2M myofibers
- German Shepherd, retrievers, and Doberman Pinscher predisposed
- Young to middle-aged dogs

Canine idiopathic polymyositis
- Large-breed dogs predisposed

Feline idiopathic polymyositis

Dermatomyositis
- Herding breeds, especially Shetland Sheepdog and Collie

Protozoal myositis
- *Toxoplasma gondii*
- *Neospora caninum Hepatozoon, Babesia, Leishmania,* or *Trypanosoma* infection

Bacterial myositis *Clostridium, Leptospira, Ehrlichia,* Rocky Mountain spotted fever

Extraocular myositis (dogs)

Feline immunodeficiency virus

Metabolic Myopathies

Glucocorticoid excess

- Hyperadrenocorticism
- Exogenous corticosteroids

Hypothyroidism

Hypoadrenocorticism

Hypokalemic polymyopathy (cat)

- Increased urinary excretion
- Decreased dietary intake

Mitochondrial myopathies

Lipid storage myopathies

Glycogen storage disorders

Malignant hyperthermia

Hyperkalemic periodic paralysis (American Pit Bull Terrier)

Inherited Myopathies

Muscular dystrophy

- Hereditary Labrador Retriever muscular dystrophy
- Also German Shorthaired Pointer, Rottweiler, others
- Maine Coon, Siamese, Devon Rex, Sphynx, others

Myotonia

- Chow Chow, Staffordshire Bull Terrier, Labrador Retriever, Rhodesian Ridgeback, Great Dane, others

Malignant hyperthermia

- Hypermetabolic disorder of skeletal muscle
- Genetic defect in intracellular calcium homeostasis

Inherited myopathy of Great Danes

Centronuclear myopathy

- Labrador Retriever

Episodic/Exercise-induced collapse

- Labrador Retriever

Exertional rhabdomyolysis

Neurologic Examination

Components

Mental State

Normal

Depression

Stupor

Coma

Agitation

Delirium

Posture

Normal, upright
Head tilt
Wide-based stance
Recumbent
Extensor posturing
Opisthotonus
Pleurothotonus

Gait

Proprioceptive deficits
Paresis
Circling
Ataxia
Dysmetria
Lameness

Postural Reactions

Conscious proprioception
Hopping
Wheelbarrowing
Hemiwalking
Extensor postural thrust

Muscle Tone

Atrophy
Decreased muscle tone (lesions of lower motor
neurons)
Increased muscle tone (lesions of upper motor
neurons)
Schiff-Sherrington posture (increased muscle tone and
hyperextension of thoracic limbs)

Spinal Reflexes

Absent, depressed, normal, or exaggerated
Thoracic limb withdrawal (sixth cervical [C6], C7, C8,
first thoracic [T1])
Biceps (C6-C8) and Triceps (C7-T2) reflexes
Patellar (fourth lumbar [L4], L5, L6)
Pelvic limb withdrawal (L6, L7, first sacral [S1])
Sciatic (L6, L7, S1)
Cranial tibial (L6, L7)
Perineal (S1, S2, S3, pudendal nerve)
Bulbourethral (S1, S2, S3, pudendal nerve)
Panniculus (response absent caudal to spinal cord lesion,
used at T3-L3)
Crossed extensor reflex (indicative of UMN disease)
Cutaneous trunci reflex

Sensation and Pain
Superficial pain
Deep pain
Hyperesthesia

Urinary Tract Function

Cranial Nerves

Paroxysmal Disorders Confused with Epileptic Seizures

Differential Diagnosis

Syncope (reduced cerebral blood flow)
Cardiac arrhythmias
Hypotension

Episodic Weakness
Hypoglycemia
Low blood cortisol
Electrolyte disturbances

Myasthenia Gravis

Acute Vestibular "Attacks"

Movement Disorders
Episodic falling
Scotty cramp
Head bobbing
Dyskinesias

Sleep Disorders
Narcolepsy
Cataplexy

Obsessive Compulsive Disorder

Peripheral Neuropathies

Clinical signs depend on the nerve affected and the severity of the lesion.

Differential Diagnosis

Focal Disease
Trauma
Mechanical blows
Fractures
Pressure
Stretching

Laceration
Injection of agents into nerves

Peripheral Nerve Tumors
Schwannoma
Neurofibroma
Neurofibrosarcoma
Lymphoma

Facial Nerve Paralysis
Otitis media
Trauma
Neoplasia
Foreign body (e.g., grass awn)
Nasopharyngeal polyp in cats
Hypothyroidism
Idiopathic

Trigeminal Nerve Paralysis
Bilateral, idiopathic disorder, often self-limiting
Middle-aged to older dogs, rarely cats

Idiopathic Peripheral Vestibular Disease

Hyperchylomicronemia
Leads to xanthomas in skin
May compress peripheral nerves

Ischemic Neuromyopathy
Caudal aortic thromboembolism

Generalized Chronic Polyneuropathies
Idiopathic
Metabolic disorders
- Diabetes mellitus
- Hypothyroidism
Paraneoplastic syndromes
- Insulinoma
- Other tumors
Systemic lupus erythematosus (SLE) or other immune-mediated disease
Chronic organophosphate toxicity
Ehrlichiosis

Generalized Acute Neuropathies
Acute polyradiculoneuritis ("coonhound paralysis")
Neospora polyradiculoneuritis (puppies)
Disorders of neuromuscular junction
- Botulism
- Tick paralysis
- Myasthenia gravis

Protozoal polyradiculoneuritis
Dysautonomia

Developmental/Congenital Neuropathies
Loss of motor neurons—Cairn Terrier, German Shepherd,
   English Pointer, Rottweiler, Swedish Lapland, Brittany
   Spaniel
Loss of peripheral axons—German Shepherd,
   Alaskan Malamute, Birman cat, Rottweiler, Boxer,
   Dalmatian
Schwann cell dysfunction—Golden Retriever, Tibetan
   Mastiff
Loss of sensory neuron of axon and laryngeal nerves—
   Dachshund, English Pointer, Shorthaired Pointer,
   Bouvier des Flandres, Siberian Husky
Inborn errors of metabolism
* Hyperchylomicronemia (cat)
* Hyperoxaluria type 2 (shorthaired cat)
* α-L-Fucosidosis (English Springer Spaniel)
* Atypical GM2 gangliosidosis (cat)
* Globoid cell leukodystrophy
* Niemann-Pick disease (Siamese)
* Glycogen storage disease (Norwegian forest cat)

Spinal Cord Disease

Differential Diagnosis

Acute
Trauma
Hemorrhage/coagulopathy
Infarction
Type I intervertebral disk herniation
Fibrocartilaginous embolism
Atlantoaxial subluxation

Subacute/Progressive
Discospondylitis
Noninfectious inflammatory diseases
* Corticosteroid-responsive meningitis/arteritis
* Granulomatous meningoencephalitis
* Feline polioencephalomyelitis
Infectious inflammatory diseases
* Bacterial, fungal, rickettsial, prototechal, protozoal,
   nematodiasis
Distemper myelitis
Feline infectious peritonitis (FIP) meningitis/myelitis

Chronic Progressive

Neoplasia
Type II intervertebral disk protrusion
Degenerative myelopathy
Cauda equina syndrome
Cervical vertebral malformation/malarticulation (wobbler syndrome)
Lumbosacral vertebral canal stenosis
Spondylosis deformans
Hypervitaminosis A (cats)
Dural ossification
Diffuse idiopathic skeletal hyperostosis
Synovial cyst

Progressive in Young Animals

Neuronal abiotrophies and degenerations
Metabolic storage diseases
Atlantoaxial luxation
Congenital vertebral anomalies

Congenital (Constant)

Spinal bifida
Congenital dysgenesis of Manx cats
Spinal dysraphism
Hereditary ataxia
Pilonidal, epidermoid, and dermoid cysts
Syringomyelia/hydromyelia

Spinal Cord Lesions

Localization

Cranial Cervical Lesion (C1-C5)

Upper motor neuron (UMN) signs in rear limbs
UMN signs in forelimbs

Caudal Cervical Lesion (C6-T2)

UMN signs in rear limbs
Lower motor neuron (LMN) signs in forelimbs

Thoracolumbar Lesion (T3-L3)

UMN signs in rear limbs
Normal forelimbs

Lumbosacral Lesion (L4-S3)

LMN signs in rear limbs
Loss of perineal sensation and reflexes
Normal forelimbs

Sacral Lesion (S1-S3)
Normal forelimbs
Normal patellar reflexes
Loss of sciatic function
Loss of perineal sensation and reflexes

Systemic Disease

Neurologic Manifestations

Oxygen Deprivation

Vascular Disease
Ischemia
Thromboembolic disease
Shock
Cardiac disease

Hemorrhage (anemia)
Vessel rupture secondary to hypertension
Coagulopathy
Vasculitis

Anesthetic Accidents
Hypotension
Cardiac arrhythmia
Extensive blood loss
Hypercapnia
Hypoxemia

Hypoxia
Pulmonary disease
Decreased oxygen transport
Heart failure

Hypertension

Hypoglycemia

Decreased Output or Metabolism
Primary liver disease
Malnutrition
Thiamine deficiency

Increased Uptake
Hyperinsulinemia
Islet cell tumors
Insulin overdose

Non–Islet Cell Neoplasia
Hepatoma
Leiomyoma

Excessive Metabolism
Sepsis
Breed or activity-related

Increased Uptake of Amino Acids by Extrahepatic Tissues

Water and Ionic Imbalances
Water
Hypoosmolar States (Retention of Free Water)
Hyponatremia

Hyperosmolar States (Loss of Free Water)
Hypernatremia (diabetes insipidus)
Hyperglycemia (diabetes mellitus)

Ions (Excess or Deficiency)
Calcium
Potassium

Endogenous Neurotoxins
Renal Toxins

Hepatoencephalopathy

Endocrine Disease
Adrenal
Hyperadrenocorticism
Hypoadrenocorticism

Adrenergic Dysregulation
Pheochromocytoma

Thyroid
Hypothyroidism
• Myxedema
• Neuromyopathy
Thyrotoxicosis
• Hyperthyroidism
• Iatrogenic

Exogenous Neurotoxins
Plant toxins
Sedative depressant drugs (e.g., antiepileptic drugs)
Heat stroke

Remote Neurologic Manifestations of Cancer
Metastasis to the nervous system
Vascular accidents and infection
Adverse effects of therapy
Paraneoplastic syndromes

Vestibular Disease

Clinical Findings

Central and Peripheral Vestibular Disease

Head tilt to side of lesion
Circling/falling/rolling to side of lesion
Vomiting, salivation
Incoordination
Ventral strabismus on side of lesion (±)
Nystagmus, fast phase away from lesion
Nystagmus may intensify with changes in body position.

Peripheral Vestibular Disease

Nystagmus is horizontal or rotatory.
No change in nystagmus direction with changes in head
position
Postural reactions and proprioception normal
Concurrent Horner syndrome, cranial nerve VII paralysis
with middle/inner ear involvement; other cranial
nerves normal

Central Vestibular Disease

Nystagmus horizontal, rotatory, or vertical
Nystagmus direction may change direction with change
in head position.
Abnormal postural reactions and proprioception may be
seen on side of lesion.
Multiple cranial nerve deficits may be seen.

Paradoxical Vestibular Syndrome (Cerebellar Lesion)

Head tilt and circling away from side of lesion
Fast phase nystagmus toward the lesion
May exhibit vertical nystagmus
Abnormal postural reactions on side of lesion
± Multiple cranial nerve deficits on side of lesion
± Hypermetria, truncal sway, and head tremor

Ocular Disorders

Anisocoria

Differential Diagonosis

Nonneurologic Causes of Anisocoria

Conditions That Cause Miosis

- Anterior uveitis
- Corneal ulcers and lacerations (reflex miosis mediated by trigeminal nerve)

Conditions That Cause Mydriasis

- Iris atrophy
- Iris hypoplasia
- Glaucoma
- Iridal tumors (e.g., melanoma) that infiltrate iridal musculature
- Unilateral retinal disease (e.g., retinal detachment)
- Severe chorioretinitis that affects a larger area on one eye than the other
- Unilateral optic neuritis or optic nerve neoplasia
- Orbital neoplasia, retrobulbar abscess, cellulitis

Pharmacologic Causes of Anisocoria

Drugs That Cause Miosis (usually agents used for management of glaucoma)

- Pilocarpine
- Demecarium bromide
- Synthetic prostaglandins such as latanoprost

Drugs That Cause Mydriasis

- Tropicamide, atropine

- Ocular contact with toxins like jimsonweed *(Datura stramonium)*
- Ocular decongestants like phenylephrine

Neurologic Causes of Anisocoria

Afferent Lesions

Anisocoria is reduced or abolished in darkness as both pupils dilate. This is because the stimulus producing the anisocoria, light causing constriction of the normal pupil, is eliminated.

- Unilateral retinal or prechiasmal optic nerve lesion
- Unilateral optic tract lesion
- Optic chiasm lesion

Efferent Lesions

Parasympathetic efferent lesions (In dogs, preganglionic efferent nerves are purely parasympathetic and postganglionic nerves are mixed. In cats both nerves are purely parasympathetic.)

- Lesions of the nucleus of CN III, the preganglionic fibers, or the ganglion itself

Sympathetic efferent lesions (Loss of sympathetic tone to the eye is known as Horner syndrome, is always ipsilateral to lesion, and features miosis, ptosis, protrusion of the third eyelid, and enophthalmos.)

- Head, neck, or chest trauma
- Brachial plexus avulsion
- Intracranial, mediastinal, or intrathoracic neoplasia
- Otitis media/interna
- Injury to the ear during ear flushing
- Idiopathic (Golden Retriever and Collie may be predisposed.)

Blindness, Acute

Differential Diagnosis, Dogs and Cats

Cornea

Edema (glaucoma, trauma, endothelial dystrophy, immune-mediated keratitis, neurotropic keratitis, anterior uveitis)

Melanin (entropion, ectropion, lagophthalmos, facial nerve paralysis, keratoconjunctivitis sicca, pannus)

Cellular infiltrate (bacterial, viral, fungal)

Vascular invasion (exposure keratitis)

Fibrosis (scar formation)

Dystrophy (lipid, genetic)

Symblepharon (conjunctiva adhered to cornea)

Aqueous Humor

Fibrin (anterior uveitis: many etiologies)

Hyphema (trauma, coagulopathies, neoplasia, systemic hypertension, retinal detachment)

Hypopyon (immune-mediated, lymphoma, systemic fungal infection, toxoplasmosis, FIP, prototheocosis, brucellosis, bacterial septicemia)

Lipemic (hyperlipidemia with concurrent blood-aqueous barrier disruption [uveitis])

Lens

Cataracts (genetic, diabetes, retinal degeneration, hypocalcemia, electric shock, chronic uveitis, lens luxation, metabolic, toxic, traumatic, nutritional)

Vitreous

Hemorrhage (trauma, systemic hypertension, retinal detachment, neoplasia, coagulopathy)

Hyalitis (numerous infectious agents, penetrating injury)

Retina

Retinopathy (glaucoma, sudden acquired retinal degeneration [SARD], progressive retinal atrophy, central progressive retinal atrophy, feline central retinal atrophy, toxicity, taurine deficiency in cats, vitamin E deficiency in dogs, enrofloxacin toxicity in cats)

Chorioretinitis (systemic mycoses, ehrlichiosis, RMSF, canine distemper, toxoplasmosis, FIP, prototheocosis, brucellosis, bacterial septicemia, intraocular larval migrans, neoplasia)

Retinal detachment (neoplasia, retinal dysplasia, hereditary/congenital, exudative/transudative disorders such as systemic hypertension or infection-induced inflammatory disease)

Lesions that Prevent Transmission of the Image (optic nerve disease)

Viruses (canine distemper, feline infectious peritonitis [FIP])

Systemic diseases (neoplasia, traumatic avulsion of optic nerve, granulomatous meningoencephalitis, hydrocephalus, optic nerve hypoplasia, immune-mediated optic neuritis, systemic mycoses)

Lesions that Prevent Interpretation of the Visual Message

Canine distemper, FIP, toxoplasmosis, granulomatous meningoencephalitis, systemic mycoses, trauma, heat stroke, hypoxia, hydrocephalus, hepatoencephalopathy, neoplasia, storage diseases, postictal, meningitis

Corneal Color Changes

Diagnostic Tests

Red (blood vessels)
- Mechanism is chronic irritation
- Fluorescein stain, Schirmer tear test (STT), palpebral and corneal reflexes

"Fluffy" Blue (stromal edema)
- Mechanisms are endothelial or epithelial dysfunction
- Fluorescein stain, intraocular pressure (IOP), flare, check for lens luxation

"Wispy" Gray (stromal scar)
- Mechanism is previous (inactive) inflammation
- Fluorescein stain

"Sparkly" White (lipid/mineral accumulation)
- Mechanisms are dystrophy, degeneration, or hyperlipidemia
- Flourescein stain, systemic lipid analysis

Black (pigmentation)
- Mechanism is chronic irritation
- Fluorescein stain, STT

"Punctate" Tan (keratinic precipitates or staphyloma)
- Mechanism is uveitis
- IOP, flare, systemic disease testing

Yellow-Green (inflammatory cell infiltration)
- Inflammation (usually septic)
- Fluorescein stain, cytology, culture and sensitivity testing, polymerase chain reaction (PCR)

Eyelids and Periocular Skin

Differential Diagnosis

Infectious Blepharitis
Bacterial Blepharitis
- Usually *Staphylococcus* spp.
- External hordeolum or stye—infection of the glands of Zeis or Moll
- Internal hordeolum—infection of the meibomian glands
- Chalazion—meibomian secretions thicken and obstruct the duct, leading to glandular rupture and lipogranuloma formation

Fungal Blepharitis
- Dermatophytes *(Microsporum canis, Microsporum gypseum, Trichophyton mentagrophytes)*
- *Malassezia pachydermatitis*—most dogs with *Malassezia* dermatitis have concurrent dermatoses, in cats *Malassezia* infection is linked to systemic disease like diabetes, retroviral infection, internal neoplasia

Parasitic Blepharitis
- Demodecosis
- Feline herpetic ulcerative dermatitis

Allergic Blepharitis
- Atopic dermatitis
- Cutaneous adverse food reaction (food allergy)

Metabolic/Nutritional Blepharitis
- Zinc-responsive dermatosis
- Superficial necrolytic dermatitis (hepatocutaneous disease)

Immune-Mediated Blepharitis
- Pemphigus foliaceus
- Pemphigus erythematosus
- Systemic lupus erythematosus
- Erythema multiforme

Iatrogenic Blepharitis
- Adverse reactions to topical medications

Pigmentary Changes Involving the Eyelid
- Lentigo simplex of orange cats (black macules, not pathogenic)
- Vitiligo (hypopigmentation)
- Uveodermatologic (Vogt-Koyanagi-Harada-like) syndrome (leukoderma)

Neoplastic Blepharitis
- Meibomian gland adenoma
- Papillomas
- Squamous cell carcinoma
- Lymphosarcoma
- Mast cell tumor

Miscellaneous Eyelid Diseases
- Juvenile sterile granulomatous dermatitis and lymphadenitis/juvenile cellulitis (puppy strangles)
- Canine reactive histiocytosis

- Entropion
- Ectropion
- Distichiasis
- Trichiasis

Nonhealing Corneal Erosions (Ulcers) in Dogs

Causes

Establish underlying cause of impaired wound healing.
- Mechanical trauma from lid masses
- Entropion
- Foreign bodies
- Secondary infection
- Corneal exposure caused by lid paralysis
- Exophthalmos
- Buphthalmos
- Tear film abnormalities
- Conformational abnormalities resulting in lagophthalmos
- Corneal edema
- Distichiasis
- Facial fold irritation of cornea

Spontaneous Chronic Corneal Epithelial Defects (SCCEDs)—also called *indolent erosions/ulcers* or *boxer erosions/ulcers*
- Middle-aged dogs
- Boxers predisposed
- Likely instigated by superficial trauma
- Dogs with diabetes mellitus predisposed
- Rim of loose epithelium surrounds corneal defect
- No loss of stromal substance (stromal loss indicates more severe process, typically infection)
- Blepharospasm/epiphora
- Neovascularization may be delayed compared with healing corneal ulcers.

Bullous Keratopathy

Ocular Manifestations of Systemic Diseases

Surface Ocular Disease

Eyelids
Immunosuppressive disorders may predispose to meibomian gland infection with *Demodex* or *Staphylococcus* spp.
Eyelids have mucocutaneous junction; affected by autoimmune disorders such as systemic lupus

erythematosus (SLE) and pemphigoid diseases; also may
be affected by uveodermatologic syndrome and vasculitis

Altered lid position, cranial nerve III or VII dysfunction

Horner syndrome: decreased sympathetic tone causing
enophthalmos with third eyelid protrusion, ptosis,
and miosis; often idiopathic; may be seen with
disease of brain, spinal cord, brachial plexus, thorax,
mediastinum, neck, temporal bone, tympanic bulla,
or orbit

Conjunctivitis

May reflect disease of deeper ocular structures

Good location to detect pallor, cyanosis, icterus

Feline herpesvirus type 1 (FHV-1) and *Chlamydophila felis*
are primary pathogens of the conjunctiva.

Cornea/Sclera

Creamy pink discoloration of cornea may be seen with
lymphoma.

Corneal lipidosis appears similar; it may be secondary
to hyperlipidemia from hypothyroidism, hyperadrenocorticism, diabetes mellitus, and familial
hypertriglyceridemia.

Keratoconjunctivitis Sicca

Most cases are caused by lymphoplasmacytic
dacryoadenitis.

Rarely seen with xerostomia (Sjögren-like syndrome)

Possible causes include drug therapy, atropine, sulfa
drugs, etodolac, and anesthetic agents.

Others causes include canine distemper, FHV-1, and
dysautonomia.

Uveal Tract, Lens, Fundus

Uveal Tract

Hyphema or Hemorrhage

Hypertension, rickettsial disease, trauma,
coagulopathy, lymphoma, metastatic neoplasia

Protein or Fibrin Deposition

Trauma, feline infectious peritonitis (FIP),
uveodermatologic syndrome, lens capsule rupture,
rickettsial disease

Cellular (Hypopyon) or Granulomatous Infiltrates

Trauma, lymphoma, metastatic neoplasia,
uveodermatologic syndrome, algae or yeast,
lens capsule rupture, FIP, systemic mycoses,
toxoplasmosis

Other infectious agents associated with uveal tract disease include feline immunodeficiency virus (FIV), feline leukemia virus (FeLV), mycobacteria, FHV-1, *Bartonella* spp., *Ehrlichia* spp., *Leishmania donovani, Rickettsia rickettsii, Brucella canis, Leptospira* spp., and canine adenovirus.

Iris Abnormalities (Papillary Changes)
Anisocoria with FeLV
Miosis with Horner syndrome
Mydriasis with dysautonomia

Lens
Cataracts
Most common cause in dogs is hereditary.
Cataracts are frequent complication of diabetes mellitus.
Uveitis may also cause cataracts (most common cause in cats).
Other causes include hypocalcemia (hypoparathyroidism), electric shock, lightning strike, altered nutrition (e.g., puppies fed milk replacer).

Lens Luxation/Subluxation
Most often secondary to severe intraocular disease (uveitis)
May be primary in terriers

Fundus
Usually affected by diseases that extend from the uveal tract (*see* previous section) or from central nervous system (immune-mediated diseases such as granulomatous meningoencephalitis or neoplasia of CNS).

Papilledema
Optic nerve edema without hemorrhage, exudates, or blindness
Seen with increased intracranial pressure

Taurine Deficiency
Retinal degeneration
May also cause dilated cardiomyopathy

Retinal Visualization
Allows assessment of systemic condition including anemia (attenuated, pale vessels), hyperlipidemia (creamy orange hue to vessels), hyperviscosity (increased vessel tortuosity)

Systemic Hypertension
Causes extravasation of blood into retina, choroid, or subretinal space

Ocular Neoplasia

Orbital Neoplasia (presents as exophthalmos, strabismus, protrusion of the third eyelid, epiphora, and exposure keratitis)

- Osteosarcoma
- Multilobular osteosarcoma
- Fibrosarcoma
- Invasion of orbit by neoplasms of surrounding structures such as nose, sinuses, oral cavity, and orbital glands (nasal adenocarcinoma most commonly)
- Cats are more likely to have invasion of orbit from surrounding structures (fibrosarcoma, undifferentiated sarcoma, adenocarcinoma, lymphoma). Rarely see primary orbital neoplasia (squamous cell carcinoma, melanoma)

Adnexal Neoplasia (eyelid neoplasia common in dogs and rare in cats)

- 90% of eyelid tumors are benign (meibomian adenomas, melanomas, papillomas most commonly).
- Less common adnexal tumors include histiocytoma, malignant melanoma, adenocarcinoma, basal cell carcinoma, mast cell tumor, squamous cell carcinoma, hemangiosarcoma.
- Squamous cell carcinoma is the most common eyelid tumor in cats. Associated with sun exposure in cats that lack periocular pigmentation.

Surface Ocular Neoplasia (tumors of the conjunctiva, third eyelid, cornea)

- Dermoid
- Epibulbar or limbal melanocytoma
- Conjunctival neoplasia: hemangioma, hemangiosarcoma, mast cell tumor, lymphoma, squamous cell carcinoma, papilloma
- Third eyelid neoplasia: adenocarcinoma (most common), hemangiosarcoma, lobular adenoma, squamous cell carcinoma, melanoma

Intraocular Neoplasia (present with glaucoma, hyphema, corneal edema, buphthalmos, dyscoria, uveitis, retinal detachment, blindness)

- Anterior uveal melanoma (most common), 82% are benign in dogs, poorer prognosis in cats
- Other primary tumors of dogs include ciliary body adenocarcinoma and medulloepithelioma.
- Other primary tumors of cats include posttraumatic sarcoma and lymphoma.

Red Eye

Differential Diagnosis

Erythema of Primarily Conjunctival Vessels
- Corneal ulceration
- Eyelid abnormalities
- Dacryocystitis
- Cilia abnormalities
- Keratoconjunctivitis sicca
- Allergic conjunctivitis
- Bacterial or fungal keratitis
- Orbital disease

Erythema of Primarily Episcleral Vessels
- Anterior uveitis (low intraocular pressure)
- Glaucoma (high intraocular pressure)

Focal Erythema
Masses
- Prolapse of the gland of the third eyelid
- Neoplasia
- Episcleritis
- Nodular granulomatous episcleritis
- Granulation tissue

Hemorrhage
- Trauma
- Systemic disease (vasculitis, coagulopathy)

Retinal Detachment

Differential Diagnosis

Three Main Mechanisms—exudative, associated with retinal tears (rhegmatogenous), or traction pulling on retina
- Trauma—penetrating injuries such as animal bites, projectiles, or foreign bodies may result in retinal tears or induce intraocular hemorrhage, inflammation, or vitreous infection with subsequent traction retinal detachment. Typically unilateral, although strangulation can lead to bilateral retinal detachment
- Ocular anomalies such as severe retinal dysplasia, optic nerve colobomas, vitreous abnormalities, and retinal nonattachment (developmental failure of the two retinal layers to unite)
- Later-onset ocular anomalies such as cataracts and vitreous degeneration may lead to rhegmatogenous RD, especially

with rapid-forming or hypermature cataracts that lead to lens-induced uveitis.
- Hypertension is most often related to renal disease but may also be seen with hyperthyroidism and pheochromocytoma.
- Hyperviscosity—severe hyperlipidemia, hyperglobulinemia, polycythemia
- Neoplasia—most commonly due to multiple myeloma (hyperproteinemia and hyperviscosity) and lymphoma (infiltration of retina and choroid). Large intraocular tumors may induce traction retinal detachment.
- Chorioretinitis, retinochoroiditis
  - Bacteria (leptospirosis, brucellosis, bartonellosis
  - Rickettsia (ehrlichiosis, Rocky Mountain spotted fever)
  - Fungal (aspergillosis, blastomycosis, coccidioidomycosis, histoplasmosis, cryptococcosis)
  - Algae (geotrichosis, prototothecosis)
  - Viral (canine distemper virus, FIP)
  - Secondary to retroviral infection (FeLV, FIV by predisposing to lymphosarcoma or an opportunistic infection like toxoplasmosis)
  - Parasitic (causes smaller areas of detachment—larval migrans of strongyles, ascarids, or *Baylisascaris* larvae. Toxoplasmosis, leishmaniasis, neospora, babesiosis.
- Immune-mediated disease—causes vasculitis with or without chorioretinitis
  - Systemic lupus erythematosus
  - Uveodermatologic syndrome
  - Granulomatous meningoencephalitis
- Toxic—trimethoprim/sulfa or ethylene glycol in dogs, griseofulvin in cats
- Idiopathic

Uveitis

Differential Diagnosis in the Dog(d) and Cat(c)

Systemic Infection

Bacterial
- Bacteremia or septicemia (d, c)
- Bartonellosis (d, c)
- Leptospirosis (d)
- Borreliosis (d)
- Brucellosis (d)

Rickettsial
- Ehrlichiosis (d, c)
- Rocky Mountain spotted fever (d)

Viral
- Canine adenovirus-1 (d)
- Feline leukemia virus (c)
- Feline immunodeficiency virus (c)
- Feline infectious peritonitis (c)

Mycotic
- Blastomycosis (d, c)
- Histoplasmosis (d, c)
- Coccidiomycosis (d, c)
- Cryptomycosis (d, c)
- Aspergillosis (d)

Algal
- Protothecosis

Parasitic
- Aberrant nematode larval migration
- *Toxocara* (ocular larval migrans) (d, c)
- *Dirofilaria* larvae (d)

Protozoan
- Toxoplasmosis (d, c)
- Leishmaniasis (d, c)

Immune-Mediated uveitis
- Idiopathic anterior uveitis (d, c)
- Lens-induced uveitis (d, c)
- Canine adenovirus vaccine reaction (d)
- Uveodermatologic syndrome (d) (primarily Akita and Arctic breeds)
- Pigmentary uveitis (d) (primarily Golden Retrievers)

Neoplasia
- Primary (d, c)
- Metastatic (most commonly lymphoma) (d, c)

Metabolic
- Diabetes mellitus (lens-induced uveitis) (d)
- Hyperlipidemia (d)

Trauma
- Blunt or sharp (d, c)

Miscellaneous Causes of Blood/Eye Barrier Disruption
- Hyperviscosity syndrome (d, c)
- Hypertension (d, c)
- Scleritis (d)
- Ulcerative keratitis (d, c)

Toxicology

Chemical Toxicoses
Plant Toxicoses
Venomous Bites and Stings

Chemical Toxicoses

Toxicants

Kerosene, Gasoline, Mineral Seal Oil, Turpentine, Others
Pulmonary, central nervous system (CNS), and gastro-intestinal (GI) signs: may lead to hepatotoxicity, renal toxicity, and cardiac arrhythmias

Naphthalene (Mothballs)
Vomiting, lethargy, seizures, acute Heinz body hemolytic anemia, methemoglobinemia, hemoglobinuria, renal failure

Ethanol, Methanol (Wood Alcohol)
CNS depression, behavioral changes, ataxia, hypothermia, respiratory and cardiac arrest

Ethylene Glycol
Early intoxication: ataxia, progresses to oliguric renal failure with renomegaly, vomiting, hypothermia, coma, and death

Soaps and Detergents
GI irritants

Household Corrosives
Toilet bowl cleansers, calcium/lime/rust removers, drain cleaners, oven cleaners, bleaches

Propylene Glycol
Ataxia, CNS depression

Phenol Products (Household Cleaners)
Cats particularly sensitive; hepatic and renal damage, ataxia, weakness, tremors, coma, seizures, respiratory alkalosis

Anticoagulant Rodenticides
Petechiae, ecchymosis, weakness, pallor, respiratory distress, CNS depression, hematemesis, epistaxis, melena, ataxia, paresis, seizures, sudden death

Zinc Phosphate

Anorexia, lethargy, weakness, abdominal pain, vomiting early after ingestion, progresses to recumbency, tremors, seizures, cardiopulmonary collapse, death

Cholecalciferol (Vitamin D) Rodenticides and Medications

Anorexia, CNS depression, vomiting, muscle weakness, constipation, bloody diarrhea, polyuria/polydipsia

Bromethalin Rodenticides

High-dose exposure: muscle tremors, hyperexcitability, vocalization, seizures, hyperesthesia, vomiting, dyspnea

Pyrethrin and Pyrethroid Insecticides

CNS depression, hypersalivation, muscle tremors, vomiting, ataxia, dyspnea, anorexia, hypothermia, hyperthermia, seizures, rarely death

Organophosphate and Carbamate Insecticides

Muscarinic signs (salivation, lacrimation, bronchial secretion, vomiting, diarrhea) and nicotinic signs (muscle tremors, respiratory paralysis), mixed signs (CNS depression, seizures, miosis, hyperactivity)

2,4-Dichlorophenoxyacetic Acid

Vomiting, diarrhea; greater exposure may cause CNS depression, ataxia, and hindlimb myotonia.

Lead (Paints, Batteries, Linoleum, Solder, Plumbing Supplies, Fishing Weights)

High-level exposure: vomiting, abdominal pain, anorexia, diarrhea, megaesophagus
CNS signs, behavioral changes, hysteria, ataxia, tremors, opisthotonos, blindness, seizures

Zinc

Acute ingestion: vomiting, CNS depression, lethargy, diarrhea
Chronic exposure: anorexia, vomiting, diarrhea, CNS depression, pica, hemolysis, regenerative anemia, spherocytosis, inflammatory leukogram, icterus, renal failure

Iron

Vomiting, diarrhea, abdominal pain, hematemesis, melena; rarely, progresses to multisystemic failure

Plant Toxicoses

Plants That Cause Hemolysis

Onion

Plants That Affect the Cardiovascular System

Cardiac glycoside toxicity: bradycardia with first-, second-, or third-degree atrioventricular (AV) block, ventricular arrhythmias, asystole, and sudden death; also see gastrointestinal (GI) signs

Common oleander *(Nerium oleander)*
Yellow oleander *(Thevetia peruviana)*
Foxglove *(Digitalis purpurea)*
Lily of the valley *(Convallaria majalis)*
Kalanchoe *(Bryophyllum* spp.)

Azalea *(Rhododendron* spp.): weakness, hypotension, dyspnea, respiratory failure, GI signs

Yew *(Taxus* spp.): conduction disturbances, bradycardia, GI signs, weakness, seizures; poor prognosis once signs are seen

Plants Affecting the Gastrointestinal System

Oxalate-containing plants: gastric and ocular irritants

Dumbcane *(Dieffenbachia* spp.)
Philodendron *(Philodendron* spp.)
Peace lily *(Spathiphyllum* spp.)
Devil's ivy *(Epiprennum aureum)*
Rhubarb leaves *(Rheum* spp.)

Philodendron may cause renal and central nervous system (CNS) signs in cats.

Chinaberry tree *(Melia azedarach):* vomiting, diarrhea, abdominal pain, hypersalivation, may progress to CNS signs and death

Cycad palms *(Cycas* spp.) or sago palms *(Macrozamia* spp.): vomiting, diarrhea, followed by lethargy, depression, liver failure, and death (dogs)

English ivy *(Hedera helix):* GI irritation, profuse salivation, abdominal pain, vomiting, diarrhea

Castor bean plant *(Ricinus communis):* ricin is among the most deadly poisons in the world; severe abdominal pain, vomiting, diarrhea, seizures, cerebral edema; prognosis for recovery is poor once clinical signs develop.

Holly *(Ilex* spp.), poinsettia *(Euphorbia pulcherrima),* mistletoe *(Phoradendron flavescens):* mild GI irritation, occasionally diarrhea, more serious effects with mistletoe

Amaryllis, jonquil, daffodil (family Amaryllidaceae), tulip (family Liliaceae), iris (family Iridaceae): ingestion of bulb associated with mild to moderate gastroenteritis

Autumn crocus *(Colchinum autumnale)*, glory lily *(Gloriosa* spp.): colchicine, vomiting, diarrhea, abdominal pain, hypersalivation progressing to depression, multiple organ system collapse and death

Solanaceae family: tomato, eggplant, deadly or black nightshade, Jerusalem cherry-solanine, gastric irritant; may cause CNS depression and cardiac arrhythmias; nightshade can also contain belladonna.

Mushrooms: amanitine poisoning *(Amanita virosa, Amanita phalloides, Conocybe filaris)*, orellanine poisoning *(Cortinarius orellanus, Cortinarius rainierensis)*, monomethylhydrazine *(Gyromitra esculenta)*—severe hepatic disease; survivors of hepatic phase may succumb to renal tubular necrosis.

Plants Affecting the Neurologic System

Tobacco *(Nicotiana tabacum):* vomiting, CNS involvement, cardiac involvement

Hallucinogenic plants: psilocybins or "magic mushrooms," marijuana *(Cannabis sativa)*, jimsonweed *(Datura stramonium)*, thorn apple *(Datura metaliodyl)*, blue morning glory *(Ipomoea violacea)*, nutmeg *(Myristica fragrans)*, peyote (family Cactaceae)

Nettle toxicity (family Urticaceae): hunting dogs, toxins contained in needles (histamine, acetylcholine, serotonin, formic acid), salivation, vomiting, pawing at mouth, tremors, dyspnea, slow and irregular heartbeat

Macadamia nuts: locomotor disturbances, tremors, ataxia, weakness

Yesterday, today, tomorrow *(Brunfelsia* spp.)

Plants Affecting the Renal System

Easter lily *(Lilium longiflorum)* and daylily *(Hemerocallis* spp.), possibly other lilies: toxic to cats, vomiting, depression, anorexia, leading to acute renal failure, poor prognosis without early treatment

Raisins/grapes: acute renal failure

Plants Causing Sudden Death

Seeds of many fruit trees (apple, apricot, cherry, peach, plum), contain cyanogenic glycosides

Venomous Bites and Stings

Snakes, Spiders, Others

Crotalids (Pit Vipers, Rattlesnakes, Copperheads, Water Moccasins)

Enzymatic and nonenzymatic proteins, local tissue damage: localized pain, salivation, weakness, fasciculations,

hypotension, alterations in respiratory pattern, regional
lymphadenopathy, mucosal bleeding, obtundation,
convulsions, anemia, echinocytosis, stress leukogram

Elapids (Coral Snakes)
Rare envenomation, signs delayed 10-18 hours, emesis,
salivation, agitation, central depression, quadriplegia,
hyporeflexia, intravascular hemolysis, respiratory
paralysis

Latrodectus spp. (Widow Spiders)
Hyperesthesia, muscle fasciculations, cramping, somatic
abdominal pain (characteristic sign), respiratory
compromise, hypertension, tachycardia, seizures,
agitation, ataxia, cardiopulmonary collapse

Loxoscelidae (Recluse or Brown Spiders)
Cutaneous form: bull's-eye lesion, pale center with
localized thrombosis, surrounded by erythema,
develops into a hemorrhagic bulla with underlying
eschar
Viscerocutaneous form: Coombs-negative hemolytic
anemia, thrombocytopenia, disseminated intravascular
coagulation (DIC)

Tick Paralysis
Dermacentor and *Haemaphysalis* ticks, ascending paralysis,
lower motor neuron signs, megaesophagus and
aspiration pneumonia in severe cases, spontaneous
recovery a few days after tick removal

Hymenopteran Stings
Bites and stings of winged insects and fire ants
Toxic and allergic reactions (localized angioedema,
urticaria, emesis, diarrhea, hematochezia, respiratory
depression, death)

Helodermatidae Lizard (Gila Monster)
Salivation, lacrimation, emesis, tachypnea, respiratory
distress, tachycardia, hypotension, shock

Urogenital Disorders

Differentiating between Urine Marking and Inappropriate Elimination in Cats

Urine Marking

- Generally vertical surfaces (can be horizontal)
- Marking behavior (may be territorial signaling or an anxiety- or conflict-induced response)
- Most common in intact males, females in estrous
- Adults
- Urine (rarely stool)
- Doors, windows, new objects, owner's possessions, frequently used furniture

Inappropriate Elimination

- Horizontal surfaces (rarely vertical)
- Elimination behavior
- Males or females, intact or neutered
- Any age
- Urine and/or stool
- Elimination in a variety of areas

Glomerular Disease

Types, Dogs and Cats

Glomerulonephritis
  Membranoproliferative form

- Type I (mesangiocapillary)
- Type II (dense deposit disease)

Proliferative glomerulonephritis (mesangial and endocapillary)

Crescentic type (rare)

Amyloidosis

Glomerulosclerosis

Focal segmental glomerulosclerosis

Hereditary nephritis

Immunoglobulin A (IgA) nephropathy

Lupus nephritis

Membranous glomerulopathy (most common in cats)

Minimal change glomerulopathy

Differential Diagnosis for Diseases Associated with Glomerular Disease, Dogs

Infection

Bacterial
Pyelonephritis
Pyoderma
Pyometra
Endocarditis
Bartonellosis
Brucellosis
Borreliosis
Other chronic bacterial infections

Parasitic
Dirofilariasis

Rickettsial
Ehrlichiosis

Fungal
Blastomycosis
Coccidioidomycosis

Protozoal
Babesiosis
Hepatozoonosis
Leishmaniasis
Trypanosomiasis

Viral
Canine adenovirus (type I) infection

Inflammation
Periodontal disease
Chronic dermatitis

Pancreatitis
Inflammatory bowel disease
Polyarthritis
Systemic lupus erythematosus (SLE)
Other immune-mediated diseases

Neoplasia

Lymphosarcoma
Mastocytosis
Leukemia
Systemic histiocytosis
Primary erythrocytosis
Other neoplasms

Miscellaneous

Corticosteroid excess
Trimethoprim-sulfa therapy
Hyperlipidemia
Chronic insulin infusion
Congenital C3 deficiency
Cyclic hematopoiesis in gray Collies

Familial

Amyloidosis (Beagle, English Foxhound)
Hereditary nephritis (Bull Terrier, English Cocker Spaniel, Dalmatian, Samoyed)
Glomerulosclerosis (Doberman Pinscher, Newfoundland)
Glomerular vasculopathy and necrosis (Greyhound)
Mesangiocapillary glomerulonephritis (Bernese Mountain Dog)
Atrophic glomerulopathy (Rottweiler)
Proliferative and sclerosing glomerulonephritis (Soft-Coated Wheaten Terrier)

Idiopathic

Differential Diagnosis for Diseases Associated with Glomerular Disease, Cats

Infection

Bacterial

Pyelonephritis
Chronic bacterial infections
Mycoplasmal polyarthritis

Viral

Feline immunodeficiency virus (FIV)
Feline infectious peritonitis (FIP)
Feline leukemia virus (FeLV)

Inflammation
Pancreatitis
Cholangiohepatitis
Chronic progressive polyarthritis
SLE
Other immune-mediated diseases

Neoplasia
Lymphosarcoma
Leukemia
Mastocytosis
Other neoplasms

Miscellaneous
Acromegaly
Mercury toxicity

Familial

Idiopathic

Indications for Cystoscopy

- Localization of source of hematuria
- Urinary tract neoplasia
  - Determine extent and location of tumors
  - Obtain samples for cytology or histopathology
- Recurrent urinary tract infections
  - Examine for anatomic abnormalities or uroliths
  - Obtain samples for cytology, histopathology, or culture
- Urinary tract trauma
  - Examine for perforations, ruptures, and patency of urinary tract
- Urinary incontinence
  - Examine for ectopic ureters and/or urethral anomalies
  - Laser ablation of intramural ectopic ureters
  - Periurethral collagen injections for treatment of refractory urethral incompetence
- Urolithiasis
  - Confirm and remove small uroliths from bladder or urethra
  - Obtain uroliths for quantitative analysis and culture
  - Retrieve uroliths from bladder or urethra using stone forceps or stone basket
  - Fragment uroliths with laser lithotripsy
  - Fill bladder before and after voiding urohydropropulsion to remove small uroliths

Mammary Masses ·

Differential Diagnosis

- Benign mammary tumors
  - Mixed tumors (fibroadenomas)
  - Adenomas
  - Mesenchymal tumors
- Malignant mammary tumors
  - Solid carcinomas
  - Tubular adenocarcinomas
  - Papillary adenocarcinomas
  - Anaplastic carcinomas
  - Sarcomas (rare)
  - Most feline mammary tumors are adenocarcinomas
- Mammary hyperplasia
- Mastitis
- Granulomas
- Duct ectasia
- Skin tumors
- Lipomas
- Foreign bodies (e.g., BB pellets or shot may be confused with small mammary masses)

Prostatic Disease

Differential Diagnosis

Benign prostatic hyperplasia
Acute prostatitis
Chronic prostatitis
Abscess
Cyst
Prostatic neoplasia
- Adenocarcinoma most common
- Transitional cell carcinoma second most common
- Sarcomatoid carcinoma
- Primary and metastatic hemangiosarcoma
- Lymphoma

Diagnostic Evaluation

- History of lower urinary tract signs, penile discharge, hematuria, dysuria, tenesmus, obstipation, ribbon stools, stiff gait. Severe systemic signs suggest sepsis or systemic inflammation raises suspicion of acute prostatitis. Intact males are more predisposed to BPH and prostatitis.
- Digital rectal examination along with caudal abdominal palpation is a noninvasive initial screening test. The

rectum should be bilaterally symmetric, have a smooth and regular surface, have soft parenchyma, and not be painful to touch.
- Radiography of limited value for providing an actual diagnosis but may provide information about size, shape, contour, and location of the prostate. Prostatomegaly may cause dorsal displacement of the colon and cranial displacement of the urinary bladder. Mineralization with neoplasia, bacterial prostatitis, and abscessation may be apparent.
- Prostatic ultrasound is the most useful and practical imaging method. Normal prostate should have smooth borders and homogenous parenchymal pattern of moderate echogenicity. Ultrasound also offers the opportunity for guided aspirates and core biopsy sampling for culture, cytology, and histopathology.
- CT and MRI can evaluate size, shape, homogeneity of prostate and allow evaluation of intrapelvic lesions, metastatic spread, and ureteral obstruction.
- Definitive diagnosis requires cytologic, histologic, or bacteriologic evaluation of a prostate sample. Samples can be obtained using procedures such as semen collection, prostatic massage and wash, brush technique, fine needle aspiration, and biopsy.

Proteinuria in Dogs and Cats

Diagnostic Approach

- Stop use of nephrotoxic drugs.
- If proteinuria is insignificant (trace to 1+ dipstick reading and urine specific gravity > 1.035), there is no need for further workup.
- Perform urinalysis to exclude hemorrhage, infection, or inflammation as cause of proteinuria. If these conditions present, do urine culture. If these conditions are not present, do urine protein/creatinine ratio.
- Perform serum chemistry and CBC. Evaluate serum albumin and globulin.
  - Marked proteinuria ratio (UP/UC > 3) with quiet sediment and normal globulins or a polyclonal gammopathy is consistent with renal glomerular disease (glomerulonephritis, amyloidosis). Rule out causes of glomerulonephropathy such as heartworm disease, hepatozoonosis, immune-mediated diseases such as SLE, chronic infectious diseases such as borreliosis, feline leukemia virus, feline immunodeficiency virus, ehrlichiosis, other chronic inflammatory diseases, neoplasia, and hyperadrenocorticism).

- If no underlying disease found, may need renal biopsy to assess for glomerulonephritis or amyloidosis
- Proteinuria detected by precipitation testing but not dipstick or proteinuria associated with a monoclonal gammopathy may be caused by Bence Jones proteins. This requires a search for osteolytic or lymphoproliferative lesions. Ehrlichiosis may mimic myeloma. If Ehrlichia negative, protein electrophoresis in indicated. A monoclonal gammopathy suggests myeloma.

Pyelonephritis, Bacterial

Clinical Findings, Dogs and Cats

Fever
Renal pain
Leukocytosis
Anorexia
Lethargy
Cellular casts in urine sediment
Azotemia
Inability to concentrate urine
Polyuria/polydipsia
Ultrasonographic or excretory urographic abnormalities
- Renal pelvis dilatation
- Asymmetric filling of diverticula
- Dilated ureters
Bacteria in inflammatory lesions on histopathologic examination
Positive culture of ureteral urine collected by cystoscopy
Positive culture of urine obtained after rinsing bladder with sterile saline
Positive culture of urine obtained by ultrasound-guided pyelocentesis

Renal Disease

See **Glomerular Disease.**

Familial—Dogs And Cats

Amyloidosis—Beagle, English Foxhound, Shar-Pei, Abyssinian cat, Oriental shorthaired cat, Siamese cat
Renal Dysplasia—Lhasa Apso, Shih Tzu, Standard Poodle, Soft Coated Wheaten Terrier, Chow Chow, Alaskan Malamute, Miniature Schnauzer, Dutch Kooiker (Dutch decoy dog)
Fanconi syndrome (tubular dysfunction)—Basenji

Tubular dysfunction (renal glucosuria)—Norwegian Elkhound

Basement membrane disorder—Bull Terrier, Doberman Pinscher, English Cocker Spaniel, Samoyed

Membranoproliferative glomerulonephritis—Bernese Mountain Dog, Brittany Spaniel, Soft-Coated Wheaten Terrier

Primary glomerular disease—Rottweiler, Beagle, Pembroke Welsh Corgi, Newfoundland, Bullmastiff, Doberman Pinscher, Dalmatian, Bull Terrier, English Cocker Spaniel, Samoyed

Periglomerular fibrosis—Norwegian Elkhound

Polycystic kidney disease—Cairn Terrier, West Highland White Terrier, Bull Terrier, Persian cat

Multifocal cystadenocarcinoma—German Shepherd

Differential Diagnosis, Renal Tubular Disease

Cystinuria
Inherited proximal tubular defect
Many breeds of dogs including mixed breeds
Often leads to cystine calculi formation

Carnitinuria
Reported in dogs with cystinuria
May lead to carnitine deficiency and cardiomyopathy

Hyperuricosuria
Abnormal purine metabolism
- Dalmatian
- Dogs with primary hepatic disease
May lead to urate urolithiasis

Hyperxanthinuria (rare)
Seen in dogs receiving allopurinol to prevent urate uroliths
Congenital hyperxanthinuria seen in a family of Cavalier King Charles Spaniels

Renal Glucosuria
Primary renal glucouria (rare)
- Scottish Terrier, Basenji, Norwegian Elkhound, mixed breeds

Fanconi Syndrome
Inherited proximal tubular defect
Basenji most common
May lead to renal failure

Renal Tubular Acidosis
Rare tubular disorders that lead to hyperchloremic
metabolic acidosis
- Proximal renal tubular acidosis
- Distal renal tubular acidosis

Nephrogenic Diabetes Insipidus
Any renal disorder that suppresses the kidneys' response
to antidiuretic hormone (ADH)
Congenital (rare)
Acquired
- Toxic (*Escherichia coli* endotoxin)
- Drugs (glucocorticoids, chemotherapeutics)
- Metabolic disease (hypokalemia, hypercalcemia)
- Tubular injury or loss (polycystic renal disease,
  bacterial pyelonephritis)
- Medullary washout

Differentiating Acute from Chronic Renal Failure

Acute Renal Failure
- History of ischemia
- History of exposure to toxin
- Active urine sediment
- Good body condition
- Hyperkalemia (if oliguric)
- Normal to increased hematocrit
- Enlarged kidneys
- Potentially severe metabolic acidosis
- Severe clinical signs for level of dysfunction

Chronic Renal Failure
- History of previous renal disease
- History of polyuria/polydipsia
- Small irregular kidneys
- Nonregenerative anemia
- Normal to hypokalemia
- Normal to mild metabolic acidosis
- Inactive urine sediment
- Weight loss/cachexia
- Mild clinical signs for level of dysfunction

Renal Toxins in Dogs and Cats

Therapeutic Agents
Antibacterial Agents
Aminoglycosides
Sulfonamides

Nafcillin
Penicillins
Cephalosporins
Fluoroquinolones
Carbapenems
Rifampin
Tetracyclines
Vancomycin

Antifungal Agents
Amphotericin B

Antiviral Agents
Acyclovir
Foscarnet

Antiprotozoal Agents
Pentamidine
Sulfadiazine
Trimethoprim-sulfamethoxazole
Dapsone

Anthelmintics
Thiacetarsamide

Cancer Chemotherapeutics
Cisplatin/carboplatin
Methotrexate
Doxorubicin
Azathioprine

Immunosuppressive Drugs
Cyclosporine
Interleukin-2

Nonsteroidal Antiinflammatory Drugs (NSAIDs)

Angiotensin-Converting Enzyme (ACE) Inhibitors

Diuretics

Miscellaneous Agents
Dextran 40
Allopurinol
Cimetidine
Apomorphine
Deferoxamine
Streptokinase
Methoxyflurane
Penicillamine
Acetaminophen
Tricyclic antidepressants

Radiocontrast Agents

Nontherapeutic Agents
Heavy Metals
Lead
Mercury
Cadmium
Chromium

Organic Compounds
Ethylene glycol
Carbon tetrachloride
Chloroform
Pesticides
Herbicides
Solvents

Miscellaneous Agents
Mushrooms
Snake venom
Grapes/raisins
Bee venom
Lily

Pigments
Hemoglobin/myoglobin

Hypercalcemia

Causes of Acute Renal Failure in Dogs and Cats

Primary Renal Disease
Infection
Pyelonephritis
Leptospirosis
Infectious canine hepatitis

Immune-Mediated Disease
Acute glomerulonephritis
Systemic lupus erythematosus (SLE)
Renal transplant rejection

Renal Neoplasia
Lymphoma

Nephrotoxicity
Exogenous toxins
Endogenous toxins
Drugs

Renal Ischemia
Prerenal Azotemia
Dehydration/hypovolemia
Deep anesthesia
Sepsis
Shock/vasodilation
Decreased oncotic pressure
Hyperthermia
Hypothermia
Hemorrhage
Burns
Transfusion reaction

Renal Vascular Disease
Avulsion
Thrombosis
Stenosis

Systemic Diseases with Renal Manifestations
Infection
- Bacterial endocarditis
- Feline infectious peritonitis (FIP)
- Borreliosis
- Babesiosis
- Leishmaniasis

Pancreatitis
Diabetes mellitus
Hyperadrenocorticism
Hypoadrenocorticism
Hypocalcemia
Hypokalemia
Hypomagnesemia
Hyponatremia
Systemic inflammatory response syndrome (SIRS)
Sepsis
Multiple organ failure
Disseminated intravascular coagulation (DIC)
Heart failure
SLE
Hepatorenal syndrome
Malignant hypertension
Hyperviscosity syndrome
- Polycythemia
- Multiple myeloma

Urinary outflow obstruction
Envenomation

Causes of Chronic Renal Failure in Dogs and Cats

Inflammatory/infectious
- Pyelonephritis
- Leptospirosis
- Blastomycosis
- Leishmaniasis
- FIP

Familial/congenital (see p. 265)
Amyloidosis
Neoplasia
- Lymphosarcoma
- Renal cell carcinoma
- Nephroblastoma
- Tumor lysis syndrome
- Others

Nephrotoxicants (see p. 267)
Renal ischemia
Sequela of acute renal failure
Glomerulopathies (see p. 259)
Nephrolithiasis
Bilateral hydronephrosis
- Spay granulomas
- Transitional cell carcinoma at trigone obstructing both ureters
- Nephrolithiasis

Polycystic kidney disease
Urinary outflow obstruction
Idiopathic

Reproductive Disorders

Infertility—Differential Diagnosis, Canine Female

Normal Cycles

Improper breeding management
Failure to determine optimal breeding time
Female behavior
Infertile male
Elevated diestrual progesterone
- Early embryonic death
- Lesions in tubular system (vagina, uterus, uterine tubes)
- Placental lesions (brucellosis, herpes)

Normal diestrual progesterone
- Cystic follicles (ovulation failure)

Abnormal Cycles
Abnormal Estrus
Will Not Copulate
  Not in estrus
  Inexperience
  Partner preference
  Vaginal anomaly
  Hypothyroidism (possibly)

Prolonged Estrus
  Cystic follicles
  Ovarian neoplasia
  Exogenous estrogens
  Prolonged proestrus

Short Estrus
  Observation error
  Geriatric
  Ovulation failure
  Split estrus

Abnormal Interestrual Interval
Prolonged Interval
  Photoperiod (queen)
  Pseudopregnant/pregnant (queen)
  Normal breed variation
  Glucocorticoids (bitch)
  Old age
  Luteal cysts

Short Interval
  Normal (especially queen)
  Ovulation failure (especially queen)
  Corpus luteum failure
  "Split heat" (bitch)
  Exogenous drugs

Not Cycling
Prepubertal
Ovariohysterectomy
Estrus suppressants
Silent heat
Unobserved heat
Photoperiod (queen)
Intersex (bitch)
Ovarian dysgenesis
Hypothyroidism (possibly)
Glucocorticoid excess
Hypothalamic-pituitary disorder
Geriatric

Infertility—Differential Diagnosis, Canine Male

Inflammatory Ejaculate
Prostatitis
Orchitis
Epididymitis

Azoospermia
Sperm-rich fraction not collected
Sperm not ejaculated
- Incomplete ejaculation
- Obstruction
- Prostate swelling

Sperm not produced
- Endocrine
- Testicular
- Metabolic disorders

Abnormal Motility/Abnormal Morphology
Iatrogenic
Prepubertal
Poor ejaculation
Long abstinence

Abnormal Libido
Female not in estrus
Behavioral
Pain
Geriatric

Normal Libido
Improper stud management
Infertile female

Normal Libido/Abnormal Mating Ability
Orthopedic
Neurologic
Prostatic disease
Penile problem
Prepuce problem

Penis, Prepuce, and Testes Disorders— Differential Diagnosis

Acquired Penile Disorders
Penile trauma
- Hematoma
- Laceration
- Fracture of os penis

Priapism (abnormal, persistent erection)
Neoplasia
Vesicles

Warts
Ulcers

Congenital Penile Disorders
Persistent penile frenulum
Penile hypoplasia
Hypospadias (defect in closure of urethra)
Diphallia (duplication of penis)

Preputial Disorders
Balanoposthitis
- Bacteria infection
- Blastomycosis
- Canine herpesvirus
Phimosis
Paraphimosis

Testicular Disorders
Cryptorchidism
Orchitis/epididymitis
- *Mycoplasma* spp.
- *Brucella canis*
- *Blastomyces* spp.
- *Ehrlichia* spp.
- Rocky Mountain spotted fever
- Feline infectious peritonitis (FIP)
Testicular torsion
Testicular neoplasia
- Sertoli cell tumor
- Leydig cell tumor
- Seminoma

Drugs and Metabolic Disorders Affecting Male Reproduction

Glucocorticoids (hyperadrenocorticism, exogenous
glucocorticoids)
Decreased luteinizing hormone (LH), testosterone, sperm
output, seminal volume, and libido; increased sperm
abnormalities
Estrogens, androgens, anabolic steroids
Decreased LH, testosterone, and spermatogenesis
Cimetidine
Decreased testosterone, libido, and sperm count
Spironolactone, anticholinergics, propranolol, digoxin,
verapamil, thiazide diuretics, chlorpromazine, barbiturates,
diazepam, phenytoin, primidone
Decreased testosterone and libido
Progestagens, ketoconazole
Decreased testosterone

Amphoterin B, many anticancer drugs
    Decreased spermatogenesis
Diabetes mellitus
    Decreased libido and sperm count, abnormal semen
Renal failure, stress
    Decreased libido and sperm count

Ureteral Diseases

Differential Diagnosis

Vesicoureteral Reflux
Primary: 7-12 weeks old—intrinsic maldevelopment of
    ureterovesical junction, self-limiting
Secondary to lower urinary tract obstruction, urinary
    tract infection, surgical damage, neurologic disease of
    bladder, ectopic ureters

Congenital Anomalies
Ectopic ureters
Ureterocele
Ureter agenesis
Ureter duplication

Acquired Ureteral Disease
Ureteral trauma
- Blunt trauma
- Penetrating trauma
- Iatrogenic damage during surgery

Inadvertent ligation and transection during
    ovariohysterectomy
Urinoma (paraureteral pseudocyst)
Ureteral obstruction
- Intraluminal (blood clot, calculus)
- Intramural (fibrosis, stricture, neoplasia)
- Extramural (retroperitoneal mass, bladder neoplasia,
    inadvertent ligature)

Calculi (nephroliths or nephrolith fragments that have
    migrated into the ureter)
- Calcium oxalate (most common in cat)
- Struvite (both struvite and calcium oxalate are most
    common in dog)

Neoplasia
- Transitional cell carcinoma
- Leiomyoma
- Leiomyosarcoma
- Sarcoma
- Mast cell tumor

- Fibroepithelial polyp
- Benign papilloma
- Metastatic neoplasia

Urinary Tract Infection (UTI)

Clinical Findings

Lower UTI

Dysuria

Pollakiuria

Urge incontinence

Gross hematuria at end of micturition

Cloudy urine

Foul odor to urine

Small, painful, thickened bladder

Palpable urocystoliths

Pyuria

Hematuria

Proteinuria

Bacteriuria

Normal CBC

Upper UTI

Polyuria/polydipsia

Signs of systemic illness or infection

Possible renal failure

Fever

Abdominal pain

Kidneys normal to enlarged

Leukocytosis

Pyuria

Hematuria

Proteinuria

Bacteriuria

Cellular or granular casts

Decreased urine specific gravity

Acute Prostatitis or Prostatic Abscess

Urethral discharge independent of micturition

Signs of systemic illness/infection

Fever

Painful prostate or abdomen

Prostatomegaly/asymmetry

Leukocytosis (±)

Pyuria

Hematuria

Proteinuria
Bacteruria
Inflammatory prostatic cytology

Chronic Prostatitis
Recurrent UTIs
Urethral discharge independent of urination
Possible dysuria
Normal complete blood count (CBC)
Pyuria
Hematuria
Proteinuria
Bacteruria
Prostatomegaly/asymmetry

Canine Lower Urinary Tract Disease— Differential Diagnosis

Urocystoliths
Struvite (magnesium ammonium phosphate)
Calcium oxalate
Purine (urate/xanthine)
Cystine
Calcium phosphate
Silica
Compound uroliths

Urethral Obstruction
Urethroliths (*see* Urocystoliths)
Blood clots
Urethral stricture
Neoplasia
- Transitional cell carcinoma
- Prostatic adenocarcinoma
- Leiomyoma
- Leiomyosarcoma
- Prostatic adenocarcinoma
- Squamous cell carcinoma
- Myxosarcoma
- Lymphoma
- Mast cell tumor
Proliferative urethritis
Urinary bladder entrapment in perineal hernia
Trauma
- Penile fracture

Urinary Tract Trauma
Contusion (bladder or urethra)
Urethral tears

Rupture of bladder (blunt trauma, secondary to pelvic fracture, penetrating wound)
Avulsion of bladder or urethra
Penile fracture

Inflammation (Bladder or Urethra)
Bacterial UTI
Fungal UTI
Polypoid cystitis
Emphysematous cystitis
Cyclophosphamide-induced cystitis
Parasitic cystitis *(Capillaria plica)*

Feline Lower Urinary Tract Disease—Differential Diagnosis

Feline idiopathic cystitis
Urethral plug (obstructive feline idiopathic cystitis)
Urolithiasis
- Struvite
- Calcium oxalate
- Urate
- Cystine

Bacterial cystitis (less common in cats than in dogs)
Stricture
Neoplasia

Uroliths, Canine

Characteristics

Calcium Oxalate Monohydrate or Dihydrate
Radiopaque
Acidic to neutral pH
Sharp projections or smooth uroliths; calcium oxalate dihydrate uroliths may be jackstone shaped
Not associated with urinary tract infection
Calcium oxalate dihydrate crystals: square envelope shape
Calcium oxalate monohydrate crystals: dumbbell shaped

Struvite (Magnesium-Ammonium-Phosphate)
Radiopaque
Alkaline pH
Smooth to speculated if single; smooth and pyramidal in shape if multiple
Associated with infection with urease-producing bacteria *(Staphylococcus, Proteus, Ureaplasma* spp., *Klebsiella, Corynebacterium)*
"Coffin lid"–shaped crystals

Urate/Xanthine
Radiolucent to faintly radiopaque
Acidic pH
Smooth uroliths
Not associated with infection
Yellow-brown "thorn apple" (spherical) or amorphous
   crystals

Cystine
Faintly to moderately radiopaque
Acidic pH
Smooth, round uroliths; staghorn-shaped uroliths if
   nephroliths present
Not associated with infection
Hexagonal-shaped crystals

Calcium Phosphate
Radiopaque
Alkaline to normal pH for hydroxyapatite, acidic for
   brushite
Small, variably shaped uroliths for hydroxyapatite
Smooth, round or pyramidal for brushite
Not associated with infection
Amorphous phosphate crystals or thin prisms (calcium
   phosphate)

Silica
Radiopaque
Acidic to neutral pH
Jackstone-shaped uroliths
Not associated with infection
No crystals

Vaginal Discharge

Differential Diagnosis

Cornified Epithelial Cells
Normal proestrus
Normal estrus
Contamination of skin or epithelium
Ovarian remnant syndrome
Abnormal source of estrogen
• Exogenous
• Ovarian follicular cyst
• Ovarian neoplasia
Contamination of squamous epithelium

Mucus
Normal late diestrus or late pregnancy
Normal lochia
Mucometra
Androgenic stimulation

Neutrophils

Nonseptic (no microorganisms seen)
Vaginitis
Normal first day of diestrus
Metritis or pyometra

Septic
Vaginitis
Metritis
Pyometra
Abortion

Peripheral Blood
Subinvolution of placental sites
Uterine or vaginal neoplasia
Trauma to reproductive tract
Uterine torsion
Coagulopathies

Cellular Debris
Normal lochia
Abortion

Pain Diagnosis

Acute Pain Assessment

Subjective evaluation of pain in animals relies on observation and interpretation of animal behavior. Pain may be indicated by loss of normal behaviors or appearance of abnormal behaviors.

Dogs

- Restless, agitated, delirious
- Lethargic, withdrawn, dull, obtunded
- May ignore environmental stimuli
- Abnormal sleep-wake cycle, inability to sleep
- May bite, lick, or chew painful area
- Adopt abnormal body positions to cope with pain
- Ears held back, eyes wide open with dilated pupils or closed with a dull appearance
- Disuse or guarding of painful area
- Vocalization (whimper, yelp, whine, groan, yowl)
- May become more aggressive and resist handling or palpation or may become more timid and seek increased contact with caregivers

Cats

- Hide, stay to back of cage
- Behavior may be mistaken for fear or anxiety
- May sit very quietly and pain may be missed by those looking for more active signs of pain
- May continue to purr while in pain
- May growl with ears flattened
- May attempt escape
- Lack of grooming
- Hunched posture, statue-like appearance
- Reduced or absent appetite
- Tail flicking

Acute Pain Preemptive Scoring System (examples in each category)

Minor Procedures: No Pain

- Physical examination, restraint
- Radiography
- Suture removal, cast application, bandage change
- Grooming
- Nail trim

Minor Surgeries: Minor Pain

- Suturing, debridement
- Urinary catheterization
- Dental cleaning
- Ear examination and cleaning
- Abscess lancing
- Removing cutaneous foreign bodies

Moderate Surgeries: Moderate Pain

- Ovariohysterectomy, castration, caesarean section
- Feline onychectomy
- Cystotomy
- Anal sacculectomy
- Dental extraction
- Cutaneous mass removal
- Severe laceration repair

Major Surgeries: Severe Pain

- Fracture repair, cruciate ligament repair
- Thoracotomy, laminectomy, exploratory laparotomy
- Limb amputation
- Ear canal ablation

Chronic Pain Assessment

- Clinical signs of chronic pain depend on underlying cause and pathologic state.
- Range from subtle to obvious
- May see acute flareups that require changes in treatment (e.g., osteoarthritic dog that experiences acute pain after excessive strenuous activity
- Decreased activity
- Reluctance to rise or play
- Changes in sleep patterns
- Changes in appetite
- Changes in social interaction and grooming habits
- Withdrawal, aggression
- Owner observations are extremely important

PART THREE

Laboratory Values and Interpretation of Results

Note: Normal ranges are meant to provide the reader an approximation of normal. Individual laboratory values should be compared with the reference range values of the laboratory that performed the test.

Acetylcholine Receptor Antibody

Normal range:
Feline: <0.3 nmol/L
Canine: <0.6 nmol/L

Elevated in: myasthenia gravis

Note: A positive titer is diagnostic for myasthenia gravis. Negative titers occur in 10% to 20% of positive cases; therefore a negative titer does not exclude myasthenia gravis.

Activated Coagulation Time (ACT)

Normal range:
Feline: 50-75 seconds
Canine: 60-110 seconds
Screening test for intrinsic and common coagulation pathways (factors II, V, VIII, IX, X, XI, XII); may also be prolonged with severe thrombocytopenia and decreased fibrinogen.

Activated Partial Thromboplastin Time (APTT)

Normal range:
Feline: 10-25 seconds
Canine: 10-25 seconds
Determines abnormalities in the intrinsic coagulation pathway
Prolonged with deficiencies in factors VIII, IX, XI, and XII and fibrinogen; also prolonged with disseminated intravascular coagulation (DIC)
Prolonged with von Willibrand disease, acquired vitamin K deficiency, coumarin poisoning, bile insufficiency, liver failure
Severely prolonged with hemophilia A (factor VIII deficiency) and hemophilia B (factor IX)

Adrenocorticotropic Hormone (ACTH), Endogenous

Normal range:
Feline: not reported
Canine: 10-70 pg/mL

Elevated in: pituitary-dependent hyperadrenocorticism

Decreased in: iatrogenic Cushing syndrome and adrenal tumors

Adrenocorticotropic Hormone (ACTH) Stimulation Test

Normal range:

Pre-ACTH injection:
Feline: 1.0-4.5 μg/dL
Canine: 1.0-4.5 μg/dL

Post-ACTH injection:
Feline: 4.5-15.0 μg/dL (13-16 μg/dL: suggestive of hyperadreno-
    corticism, >16 μg/dL strongly suggestive)
Canine: 5.5-20.0 μg/dL (18-24 μg/dL: suggestive of hyperadre-
    nocorticism, >24 μg/dL strongly suggestive)
From 15% to 20% are false-negative results; false-positive results
    may be seen with stress or nonadrenal illness.
Pre-ACTH cortisol is in normal range, and post-ACTH cortisol
    shows little to no change with iatrogenic Cushing syndrome.
Pre-ACTH cortisol is below normal, and post-ACTH cortisol
    shows little change with hypoadrenocorticism.
Pre-ACTH and post-ACTH cortisol levels should be between 1
    and 5 μg/dL with successful Lysodren induction or while on
    maintenance Lysodren therapy.
Trilostane induction: <1.45 μg/dL, stop treatment. Restart on a
    lower dose.
1.45-5.4 μg/dL, continue on same dose.
5.4-9.1 μg/dL, continue on current dose if clinical signs well
    controlled or increase dose if clinical signs of hyperadreno-
    corticism still evident.
>9.1 μg/dL, increase initial dose.

*Note: ACTH stimulation does not differentiate pituitary-dependent hy-
peradrenocorticism from adrenal tumors. The low-dose dexamethasone
test is more diagnostic for canine Cushing syndrome.*

Alanine Aminotransferase (ALT, Formerly SGPT)

Normal range:
Feline: 10-100 IU/L
Canine: 12-118 IU/L

Elevated in: hepatocellular membrane damage and leakage
Inflammation: chronic active hepatitis, lymphocytic/plasmacytic
   hepatitis (cats), enteritis, pancreatitis, peritonitis, cholangitis,
   cholangiohepatitis
Infection: bacterial hepatitis, leptospirosis, feline infectious
   peritonitis (FIP), infectious canine hepatitis
Toxicity: chemical, heavy metals, mycotoxins
Neoplasia: primary, metastatic
Drugs
Endocrine: diabetes mellitus, hyperadrenocorticism,
   hyperthyroidism
Trauma
Hypoxia: cardiopulmonary disease, thromboembolic disease
Metabolism: feline hepatic lipidosis, storage diseases (e.g.,
   copper)
Liver lobe torsion
Hepatocellular regeneration
Cirrhosis

Decreased in: end-stage liver disease, but in most cases decreased
ALT is not significant

Albumin

Normal range:
Feline: 2.5-3.9 g/dL
Canine: 2.7-4.4 g/dL

Elevated in: dehydration (globulin and total protein should
also be increased), spurious (e.g., hemolysis, lipemia, laboratory
error), higher in adults than in juveniles

Decreased in: protein-losing nephropathy (amyloidosis,
glomerulonephritis, glomerulosclerosis), gastroenteropathy
(malabsorption, maldigestion, protein-losing enteropathy), liver
failure, malnutrition (dietary, parasitism), exudative skin disease
(vasculitis, burns, abrasions, degloving injury), neonates, external blood loss, compensatory (chronic effusions, hyperglobulinemia, multiple myeloma)

Alkaline Phosphatase, Serum (SAP or ALP)

Normal range:
Feline: 6-102 IU/L
Canine: 5-131 IU/L

Elevated in: biliary tract abnormalities (pancreatitis, bile duct neoplasia, cholelithiasis, cholecystitis, ruptured gallbladder); hepatic parenchymal disease (cholangitis/cholangiohepatitis, chronic hepatitis, nodular hypoplasia, copper storage disease, hepatic lipidosis [cats], cirrhosis, hepatic neoplasia, [lymphoma, hemangiosarcoma, hepatocellular carcinoma, metastatic carcinoma], toxic hepatitis, feline infectious peritonitis [cats]); corticosteroids; anticonvulsants (phenobarbital, primidone); endocrine disorders (diabetes mellitus, hyperadrenocorticism [dogs], hyperthyroidism [cats]); enteritis; bone isoenzyme; young dog with bone growth; osteosarcoma; osteomyelitis; ehrlichiosis; diaphragmatic hernia; passive congestion due to right heart failure; iatrogenic

Note: Almost any disorder that affects the liver can cause elevations in SAP levels.

Ammonia

Normal range:
Feline: 30-100 μg/dL
Canine: 45-120 μg/dL

Elevated in: hepatic failure (portosystemic shunt, cirrhosis); spurious (e.g., hemolysis, lipemia, laboratory error)

Note: Due to instability of samples, this test has been mostly been replaced by serum bile acids.

Amylase, Serum

Normal range:
Feline: 100-1200 U/L
Canine: 290-1125 U/L

Elevated in: pancreatitis, pancreatic neoplasia, pancreatic duct obstruction, pancreatic necrosis, enteritis, renal disease (decreased filtration of amylase)

Note: Serum amylase levels may not correlate with severity of disease. Not very sensitive or specific, especially in cats

Anion Gap

Normal range:
Feline: 12-24
Canine: 16.3-28.6

Laboratory calculation:
$[Na + K] - [Cl + HCO_3^-] =$ Anion gap

Elevated in: Metabolic acidosis from acids that do not contain chloride Metabolic acidosis with normal anion gap has an increased plasma chloride concentration and is called *hyperchloremic acidosis.*

Decreased in: hypoalbuminemia, IgG multiple myeloma

Antinuclear Antibody (ANA)

Normal range:
Reported as a titer, very laboratory dependent. Refer to your
    laboratory for normal ranges.
High positive titer, with associated clinical and clinicopathologic
    signs, supports a diagnosis of systemic lupus erythematosus
    (SLE). Many immune-mediated, inflammatory, and infectious
    diseases and neoplasms can result in low positive titers.
    Results may be false negative with chronic glucocorticoid use.

Arterial Blood Gases

Normal range:

	Canine	Feline
pH	7.35-7.45	7.36-7.44
$PaCO_2$	36-44	28-32
PaO_2	90-100	90-100
TCO_2	25-27	21-23
HCO_3^-	24-26	20-22

Blood gas interpretation:

Evaluate PaO_2

Hypoxemia: arterial oxygen tension/partial pressure (PaO_2) of less than 85 mm Hg

Emergency treatment for hypoxemia needed when PaO$_2$ is less than 60 mm Hg.

Cyanosis may be seen when PaO$_2$ is 50 mm Hg or lower, depending on hemoglobin concentration.

Potential causes of hypoxemia
Right-left shunts (patent ductus arteriosus, ventricular septal defects, intrapulmonary shunts)
Ventilation/perfusion mismatch (various pulmonary diseases)
Diffusion impairment
Hypoventilation (anesthesia, neuromuscular disease, airway obstruction, central nervous system disease, pleural space or chest wall abnormality)
Decrease in fraction of inspired oxygen (hooked up to empty oxygen tank)

Evaluate pH
Increase in pH: alkalemia (metabolic alkalosis or respiratory alkalosis)
Decrease in pH: acidemia (metabolic acidosis or respiratory acidosis)

Assess acid-base status

If acidemic:
Arterial carbon dioxide tension (PaCO$_2$) elevated: respiratory acidosis
PaCO$_2$ decreased: compensatory respiratory alkalosis
Bicarbonate (HCO$_3^-$) decreased: metabolic acidosis
HCO$_3^-$ elevated: compensatory metabolic alkalosis

If alkalotic:
PaCO$_2$ decreased: respiratory alkalosis
PaCO$_2$ elevated: compensatory respiratory acidosis
HCO$_3^-$ elevated: metabolic alkalosis
HCO$_3^-$ decreased: compensatory metabolic acidosis

Aspartate Aminotransferase (AST, Formerly SGOT)
Not considered clinically significant in the dog or cat.
Very sensitive but not very specific; significant amounts of AST found also in muscle.

Basophil Count

Normal range:
Feline: 0-150 cells/µL
Canine: 0-150 cells/µL

Elevated (basophilia) in: disorders associated with IgE production/binding (heartworm disease, atopy), inflammatory disease (gastrointestinal tract disease, respiratory tract disease), neoplasia (mast cell neoplasia, basophilic leukemia, lymphomatoid granulomatosis), associated with hyperlipoproteinemia and possibly hypothyroidism

Bicarbonate (HCO$_3^-$)

Normal range:
Feline: 20-22 mmol/L
Canine: 24-26 mmol/L

If acidemic:

Elevated in: metabolic alkalosis (with compensatory acidosis)

Decreased in: metabolic acidosis

If alkalotic:

Elevated in: metabolic alkalosis

Decreased in: metabolic acidosis (with compensatory alkalosis)

Bile Acids

Normal range:

Preprandial:
Feline and canine: 0-5.0 μmol/L

Postprandial:
Feline: 1-20.0 μmol/L
Canine: 5.0-25.0 μmol/L

Elevated in: hepatocellular disease, cholestatic disease, portosystemic shunt

Decreased in: delayed gastric emptying, malabsorption disorders, rapid intestinal transport, ileal resection
Patient must be fasted and cannot be icteric. Typically measure preprandial and 2-hour postprandial serum samples.
May also measure urine bile acids, although patients with portosystemic shunts tend to have lower urine bile acids than patients with hepatocellular disease.

Bilirubin

Normal range:
Feline: 0.1-0.4 mg/dL
Canine: 0.1-0.3 mg/dL

Elevated in: prehepatic, hemolytic anemia, cholestasis (extrahepatic [pancreatitis, cholangitis, cholecystitis, cholelithiasis, biliary neoplasia], intrahepatic [nodular hyperplasia, feline hepatic lipidosis, cholangitis/cholangiohepatitis, cirrhosis, hepatic lymphoma, acute hepatic necrosis]), duodenal perforation, ruptured gallbladder

Blood Urea Nitrogen (BUN)

Normal range:
Feline: 14-36 mg/dL
Canine: 6-25 mg/dL

Elevated in: prerenal azotemia (dehydration, hypoadrenocorticism, heart failure, shock, gastrointestinal hemorrhage, high-protein diet); increased catabolism (fever, drugs, [e.g., tetracycline]); renal failure; pyelonephritis; postrenal azotemia (urethral [obstruction, urolith, urethral tear, plant awn]; bladder [obstruction, urolith, blood clot, polyp, neoplasia, rupture])

Decreased in: diuresis (polydipsia, hyperadrenocorticism, overzealous fluid therapy, drugs [e.g., glucocorticoids], diabetes insipidus); liver failure (portosystemic shunt, cirrhosis, urea cycle enzyme deficiency); low-protein diet; malnutrition; neonates

Buccal Mucosal Bleeding Time (BMBT)

Normal range:
Feline and canine: <3 minutes
Prolonged bleeding time is a sensitive and specific indicator of diminished platelet function (e.g., severe thrombocytopenia, von Willebrand disease and uremia).

Calcium (Ca)

Normal range:
Feline: 8.2-10.8 mg/dL
Canine: 8.9-11.4 mg/dL

Elevated in: primary hyperparathyroidism; renal failure; hypo-adrenocorticism; hypercalcemia of malignancy (lymphosarcoma, apocrine gland adenocarcinoma, carcinomas [nasal, mammary gland, gastric, thyroid, pancreatic, pulmonary]; osteolytic [multiple myeloma, lymphosarcoma, squamous cell carcinoma, osteosarcoma, fibrosarcoma]); hypervitaminosis D (cholecalciferol rodenticides, plants, excessive supplementation); dehydration; granulomatous disease (systemic mycosis [blastomycosis], schistosomiasis, feline infectious peritonitis [FIP]); nonmalignant skeletal disorder (osteomyelitis, hypertrophic osteodystrophy [HOD]); iatrogenic disorder (excessive calcium supplementation, excessive oral phosphate binders); factitious disorders (serum lipemia, postprandial measurement, young animal); laboratory error; idiopathic (cats)

Decreased in: renal failure (acute and chronic); acute pancreatitis; intestinal malabsorption; primary hypoparathyroidism (idiopathic, post-thyroidectomy); puerperal tetany (eclampsia); ethylene glycol toxicity; hypoproteinemia/hypoalbuminemia; hypomagnesemia; nutritional secondary hyperparathyroidism; tumor lysis syndrome; phosphate-containing enemas; anticonvulsant medications; sodium bicarbonate administration; laboratory error

Cerebrospinal Fluid (CSF)

Normal range: Normal CSF is colorless and clear. Discoloration usually means RBCs or neutrophils are present.

Value	Canine	Feline	Cytology (%)		
WBCs ($\times10^3$/L)	$\leq$3	$\leq$2	Monocytes	87	69-100
RBCs ($\times10^6$/L)	$\leq$30	$\leq$30	Lymphocytes	4	0-27
Protein (mg/dL)	$\leq$33	$\leq$36	Neutrophils	3	0-9
			Eosinophils	0	0
			Macrophages	6	0-3

Infectious central nervous system (CNS) disease: increased white blood cells (WBCs) and protein content

Inflammatory CNS disease: increased WBCs and protein content

Brain neoplasia: normal to mild elevation of WBCs, mild elevation of protein content

Hydrocephalus, lissencephaly: normal WBCs and protein content

Degenerative myelopathy, intervertebral disk disease, polyradiculoneuritis: normal WBCs and normal to mildly increased protein content

Most common cause of RBCs in CSF is contamination during collection.

Chloride (Cl)

Normal range:

Feline: 104-128 mEq/L

Canine: 102-120 mEq/L

Often changes proportionally with sodium. In those cases it is usually easier to search for the cause of the sodium change.

Corrected Hyperchloremia (elevation of chloride disproportionate to elevation of sodium):

Excessive Loss of Sodium Relative to Chloride

Small Bowel Diarrhea (common and important)

Pseudohyperchloremia

Lipemic Samples Using Colorimetric Methods

Potassium Chloride Therapy (common and important)

Excessive Gain of Chloride Relative to Sodium

Therapy with Chloride Salts (NH_4Cl, KCl)

Total Parenteral Nutrition

Fluid Therapy (0.9% NaCl, hypertonic saline, KCl-supplemented fluids)

Salt Poisoning

Renal Chloride Retention (renal failure, renal tubular acidosis, hypoadrenocorticism, diabetes mellitus, chronic respiratory alkalosis, drug-induced [acetazolamide, spironolactone])

Exercise (endurance exercise in sled dogs, short, submaximal exercise [agility])

Corrected Hypochloremia (loss of chloride relative to sodium)

Gastrointestinal Loss

Vomiting of Stomach Contents

Selected GI diseases associated with hyperkalemia and hyponatremia in dogs without hypoadrenocorticism (trichuriasis, salmonellosis, perforated duodenal ulcer)

Renal Loss

Therapy with Thiazide or Loop Diuretics

Chronic Respiratory Acidosis

Hyperadrenocorticism

Glucocorticoid Administration

> ***Therapy with Solutions with High Sodium***
> ***Concentration Relative to Chloride***
>   Sodium Bicarbonate
>   Exercise in Racing Greyhounds

Cholesterol (CH)

Normal range:
Feline: 75-220 mg/dL
Canine: 92-324 mg/dL

Elevated in: postprandial, primary hyperlipidemia, endocrine disorders (hypothyroidism, hyperadrenocorticism, diabetes mellitus), cholestasis, dietary (high cholesterol diet), nephrotic syndrome, protein-losing nephropathy, idiopathic (Doberman Pinscher, Rottweiler)

Decreased in: liver failure, malabsorption, maldigestion, protein-losing enteropathy, portosystemic shunt, lymphangiectasia, starvation, hypoadrenocorticism

Cholinesterase

Normal range:
Feline: 500-4000 U/L
Canine: 800-4000 U/L

Decreased in: organophosphate toxicity, carbamate toxicity

Cobalamin

Normal range:
Feline: 290-1499 pg/mL
Canine: 251-908 pg/mL

Decreased in: exocrine pancreatic insufficiency, distal small intestinal disease, diffuse small intestinal disease, small intestinal bacterial overgrowth (usually combined with an increased serum folate level), hepatic disease in cats

Complete Blood Count (CBC)

Normal range:

Total white blood cell (WBC) count:
Feline: 3.5-16.0 10^3/µL
Canine: 4.0-15.5 10^3/µL

Total red blood cell (RBC) count:
Feline: 5.92-9.93 $10^6/\mu L$
Canine: 4.8-9.3 $10^6/\mu L$

Hemoglobin:
Feline: 9.3-15.9 g/dL
Canine: 12.1-20.3 g/dL

Hematocrit (packed cell volume):
Feline: 29-48%
Canine: 36-60%

Reticulocyte count:
Feline: 0-10.5% punctate or 0-1.0% aggregate
Canine: 0-1.0% aggregate

Mean corpuscular volume (MCV):
Feline: 37-61 fL
Canine: 58-79 fL

Mean corpuscular hemoglobin (MCH):
Feline: 11-21 pg
Canine: 19-28 pg

Mean corpuscular hemoglobin concentration (MCHC):
Feline: 30-38 g/dL
Canine: 30-38 g/dL

Platelet count:
Feline: 200-500 $10^3/\mu L$
Canine: 170-400 $10^3/\mu L$

Total solids:
Feline: 5.2-8.8 g/dL
Canine: 5.0-7.4 g/dL

Coombs Test

Indicates presence of antibody and/or complement on the surface of erythrocytes; supports the diagnosis of immune-mediated hemolytic anemia

Cortisol

Normal range:
Feline and canine: 1.0-4.5 μg/dL
Not a reliable indicator of disease; considerable overlap between normal patients and those with adrenal disease.

Elevated in: stress (environmental, illness), drugs (prednisone and prednisolone [may cross-react in assay], anticonvulsants), pituitary- and adrenal-dependent hyperadrenocorticism

Decreased in: drugs (suppression of adrenal function), hypoadrenocorticism

Creatine Kinase (CK, formerly CPK)

Normal range:
Feline: 56-529 U/L
Canine: 59-895 U/L

Elevated in: trauma, myositis (immune mediated, eosinophilic myositis, masticatory muscle myositis, infectious [toxoplasmosis, neosporosis], endocarditis), exertional myositis, surgery (tissue damage), nutritional (hypokalemia [polymyopathy], taurine deficiency), prolonged recumbency, intramuscular injections, pyrexia, hypothermia, postinfarct ischemia (cardiomyopathy, disseminated intravascular coagulation [DIC]), muscle ischemia secondary to status epilepticus

Creatinine

Normal range:
Feline: 0.6-2.4 mg/dL
Canine: 0.5-1.6 mg/dL

Elevated in: azotemia (prerenal, renal, postrenal, rhabdomyolysis)

Decreased in: any condition that causes decreased muscle mass

Cytologic Criteria of Malignancy

General Criteria

- Anisocytosis and macrocytosis—variation in cell size
- Hypercellularity—increased cell exfoliation due to decreased cell adherence
- Pleomorphism—variable size and shape of cells of the same type

Nuclear Criteria

- Macrokaryosis—increased nuclear size. Nuclei larger than 20 μ suggestive of neoplasia
- Inceased nucleus-to-cytoplasm ratio (N:C)—normal nonlymphoid cells have usually have a N:C of 1.3:1.8. Ratios of 1.2 or less suggestive of malignancy

- Anisokaryosis—variation in nuclear size. Especially important if the nuclei of multinucleated cells vary in size
- Multinucleation—especially important if the nuclei vary in size
- Increased mitotic figures—mitosis is rare in normal tissues
- Abnormal mitosis—improper alignment of chromosomes
- Coarse chromatin pattern—may appear ropy or cord-like
- Nuclear molding—deformation of nuclei by other nuclei within the same cell or adjacent cells
- Macronucleoli—nucleoli are increased in size (>5 μ suggestive of malignancy, for reference, RBCs are 5-6 μ in the cat and 7-8 μ in the dog
- Angular nucleoli—fusiform or have other angular shapes instead of their normal round to slightly oval shape
- Anisonucleoliosis—variation in nucleolar shape or size (especially important if the variation is within the same nucleus)

Cytologic Features of Discrete Cell (Round Cell) Tumors

Discrete Cells (Round Cells)

- Present individually in tissues, not adhered to other cells for connective tissue matrix
- Most discrete cells are of hematogenous origin.
- Aspirates of normal lymphoid tissues like spleen and lymph nodes yield discrete cells.
- Discrete cell patterns in other tissues indicate the presence of a discrete cell tumor (round cell tumor).
- Cells tend to be small to medium sized and round.

Specific Discrete Cell Tumors

Mast Cell Tumor

Highly cellular smears of predominately mast cells
- Small, red-purple intracytoplasmic granules
- Number of granules seen vary from few to so many the cytoplasma is packed with granules. Some mast cells may degranulate during aspiration. More granules in background, fewer in cells
- Anaplastic mast cell tumors may be virtually devoid of granules.

Lymphoma

Most cases of lymphoma in dogs and cats are high-grade tumors composed mostly of large blastic lymphoid cells. Cytology typically shows greater than 50% of cells are

large, blastic lymphocytes. Lymphoblasts have a high nuclear-to-cytoplasmic ratio and intensely basophilic cytoplasm.
- Low grade, well-differentiated lymphoma may yield predominately small lymphocytes. Such tumors are difficult to differentiate from normal or reactive lymphoid tissue and require biopsy and histopathology.

Canine Cutaneous Histiocytoma

Benign tumors of dendritic cell origin, common in young dogs
- Medium sized cells, round to oval nuclei that may be indented. Finely stippled chromatin with indistinct nucleoli. Moderate amount of light blue-gray cytoplasm
- Most histiocytomas regress spontaneously. The presence of small lymphocytes with these tumor cells may be seen in tumors that are regressing.

Malignant Histiocytosis/Histiocytic Sarcoma/Systemic Histiocytosis

Cytologic appearance varies from benign looking cells to populations of histiocytic cells with marked atypia.
- Common features include large discrete cells with abundant vacuolated cytoplasm, prominent cytophagia, and multinucleation. May demonstrate marked anisocytosis, anisokaryosis, and variation of nuclear:cytoplasmic ratio. Macrocytosis, karyomegaly, and large multinucleated cells are common.
- Definitive diagnosis may not be possible based on cytology alone.

Plasmacytoma

Tumors of plasma cell origin include multiple myeloma (arising primarily from bone marrow) and extramedullary plasmacytomas (usually cutaneous but may be in other sites such as GI).
- Cutaneous plasmacytomas are usually benign. GI tumors are more likely to be malignant.
- Well-differentiated plasmacytomas yield cells that resemble normal plasma cells. Small, round nuclei with deeply basophilic cytoplasm exist with or without the characteristic paranuclear clear zone. Poorly differentiated plasmacytoma cells are less distinct and demonstrate significant criteria of malignancy. Binucleate and multinucleate cells are common in both well and poorly differentiated plasmacytomas.

This and a lack of lymphoglandular bodies help differentiate these tumors from lymphosarcoma.

Transmissible Venereal Tumor

TVT cells are typically more pleomorphic than other discrete cell tumors.

- Moderate smoky to light blue cytoplasm, numerous cytoplasmic vacuoles that may also be found extracellularly. Nuclei show moderate to marked anisokaryosis and have coarse nuclear chromatin. Nucleoli may be prominent and mitotic figures are common.

Melanoma

Great imitators, cells show features of discrete cells, epithelial cells, or mesenchymal cells. Usually easily recognized due to their pigment. Individual melanin granules are rod-shaped and stain dark green to black. Cells may be heavily to sparely pigmented.

- Poorly differentiated melanomas may have sparse pigmentation and show marked criteria of malignancy.

Cytologic Features of Mesenchymal Cells

- Mesenchymal cells are cells that form connective tissue, blood vessels, and lymphatics.
- Hematopoietic cells are classified as mesenchymal cells, but because their appearance is so distinct, they are typically considered as a separate classification. Usually, discussion of mesenchymal cells implies stromal connective tissue cells.
- Cytoplasmic borders are often indistinct.
- Most connective tissues exfoliate no cells when sampled by fine needle aspiration. May see fibroblasts or fibrocytes on occasion. Reactive fibroblast may be seen in aspirates of inflamed tissue or tissues undergoing tissue repair. Reactive fibroblasts may show many criteria of malignancy, but reactive fibroblasts should be suspected when seen within a population of inflammatory cells.
- Highly cellular smears that contain predominately a pure population of mesenchymal cells are likely to indicate a mesenchymal neoplasm (sarcoma).
- Mesenchymal cells are often elongated with cytoplasm that tapers in one or more directions (referred to as *spindle cells*).
- May see elongated cells with rod-shaped nuclei to plump, minimally tapered cells with round nuclei. Neoplastic mesenchymal cell tumors may show features more consistent with epithelial or discrete cells.

Cytologic Features of Normal Epithelial Cells

- Cell-to-cell adhesion
- Although normal epithelial cells can be small to large, they can be very large and have abundant cytoplasm.
- Round to columnar to caudate in shape and have sharply defined cytoplasmic borders.
- Nuclei generally are round to oval.
- Squamous epithelial cells tend to be more individually oriented when collected by surface swabs or scrapings. As they mature, their nuclei become small and pyknotic and eventually the cell becomes anucleate.
- Respiratory and gastrointestinal cells are distinctly columnar. May show long rows of cells with nuclei lined up at the basal end. Cilia may be seen at the apical end of respiratory epithelial cells.
- Glandular epithelial cells may show evidence of tubular or acinar formation.
- Tumors of epithelial cell origin may retain characteristic features.

Cytology of Ear Canal Swabs

Bacteria

- Ear canals normally contain small amounts of bacteria.
- With bacterial otitis, large numbers of bacteria are seen free in the smear.
- Neutrophilic inflammation is sometimes seen, especially with concurrent otitis media.
- Visualization of cocci on the smear often represents *Staphylococcus* but may also be *Enterococcus* or *Streptococcus*.
- Rods most commonly indicate *Pseudomonas* followed by *Proteus* and *Escherichia coli*.

Fungi

- *Malassezia pachydermatis* is by far the most common yeast seen on ear cytologies but may be found in smaller numbers in normal ears.
- May see concurrent bacteria and yeast infection
- Yeasts overgrow when the environment is favorable.
- Rarely see *Candida* and *Microsporum*

Mites

- *Otodectes cyanotis* common primary cause of otitis (50% of cats, 5% of dogs)
- *Demodex canis* and *D. cati, Sarcoptes scabiei,* and *Notoedres cati* are infrequently seen in ear canals.

- Mites tend to wash off slides during staining. Unstained slides of ear secretions or swabs rolled in mineral oil may be better for finding mites in the ear canal. Skin scrapings of the ear pinna are best for finding *Demodex, Sarcoptes,* or *Notoedres.*

Neoplasia

- The most common benign tumors are seen in ear canal are polyps, papillomas, basal cell tumors, and ceruminous gland adenomas.
- The most common malignant tumors are ceruminous gland adenocarcinomas, squamous cell carcinomas, and other carcinomas.
- Unfortunately, neoplastic cells are rarely seen on ear cytologies.
- May only see cytologic evidence of inflammation
- Fine-needle aspiration or biopsy of otic masses is usually necessary to establish a diagnosis.

Miscellaneous

- Ceruminous otitis externa is associated with seborrheic conditions.
- Oily, yellow discharge may resemble purulent exudate, but cytology is relatively devoid of inflammatory cells.

Cytology of Nasal Swabs or Flush Specimens

Normal Findings

- *Simonsiella* spp.—large, stacked, rod-shaped bacteria, normal inhabitants of the oral cavity
- Nonkeratinized squamous epithelial cells, often with adherent bacteria, are obtained from the external nares and oropharynx.
- Ciliated pseudostratified columnar epithelial cells and mucus from nasal turbinates
- Basal epithelial cells are smaller and rounded and have dark blue cytoplasm.
- May see red blood cells from hemorrhage secondary to sampling

Infectious Agents

- Neutrophils predominate with bacterial, viral, or fungal infections.
- May also see macrophages, lymphocytes, and plasma cells
- Bacterial infection suspected when bacteria seen within neutrophils

- Because bacteria from the oral cavity are usually a pleomorphic population, monomorphic populations suggest infection.
- Bacterial infection of the nasal cavity usually is secondary to trauma, foreign bodies, viral or fungal infection, neoplasia, or oronasal fistulas.
- Intranuclear viral inclusions may be seen in epithelial nuclei with herpes infections in cats.
- Fungal hyphae may be present, may need special stains to identify. Nasal cavity fungi include *Aspergillus* spp., *Penicillium* spp., *Cryptococcus neoformans, Rhinosporidium* spp.
- Nasal mites *(Pneumonyssus caninum, Linguatula serrata). Capillaria aerophila* may be found in nasal sinuses.

Noninfectious Conditions

- Foreign bodies often consist of inhaled plant material (grass awns or foxtails).
- May lead to chronic rhinitis
- Exudates with eosinophils may be seen with inhaled allergens.
- Neoplasia of the nasal cavity is usually seen in older patients.
- Epithelial, mesenchymal tumors of nasal cavity cells, extension of oral neoplasms, or transplanted from other sites (e.g., transmissible venereal tumor)
- Most nasal tumors are epithelial in origin. Adenocarcinomas most common, followed by squamous cell carcinomas and undifferentiated carcinomas
- Mesenchymal tumors of the nasal cavity include fibrosarcomas, chondrosarcomas, osteosarcomas, hemangiosarcomas, and undifferentiated sarcomas. Do not exfoliate readily
- Round cell tumors of the nasal cavity include transmissible venereal tumors, lymphosarcomas, and mast cell tumors.

Dexamethasone Suppression Tests

Low-Dose Dexamethasone Suppression Test (LDDST)

Normal: 4-hour cortisol level suppresses to less than 50% of baseline cortisol (usually < 1.4 µg/dL), and then 8-hour cortisol remains at or near that level.

Pituitary-dependent hyperadrenocorticism (PDH):
4-hour cortisol level is suppressed to less than 50% of baseline (60% of dogs) or less than 1.4 µg/dL (25% of dogs) and an 8-hour cortisol level of less than 50% of baseline but 1.4 µg/dL or greater (25% of dogs).

Dexamethasone resistance, in which none of the above criteria is met, occurs in 40% of PDH cases.

Functional adrenal tumor (FAT):
Dexamethasone administration has no effect on cortisol levels.

High-Dose Dexamethasone Suppression Test

Differentiates PDH from FAT in cases where none of the criteria for PDH is met with the LDDST.

FAT:
8-hour cortisol level—no suppression of cortisol levels with dexamethasone administration.

PDH:
8-hour cortisol level is less than 50% of baseline cortisol or less than 1.4 µg/dL.

Disseminated Intravascular Coagulation (DIC), Diagnostic Tests

Fibrinogen: increased

Activated partial thromboplastin time (APTT): prolonged

Prothrombin time (PT): prolonged

Platelet count: decreased

Fibrin degradation products (assays for breakdown of fibrin clots): increased

D-Dimer (assays for proteolytic fragment of fibrinogen degradation): increased

Note: D-Dimer has a high negative predictive value. A negative test reliably rules out DIC.

Eosinophil Count

Normal range:
Feline: 0-1000 cells/µL
Canine: 0-1200 cells/µL

Eosinophils:

Elevated (eosinophilia) in: parasitic disorders (hookworm, dirofilariasis, dipetalonemiasis, fleas, filaroides, aelurostrongylosis, roundworms, paragonimiasis, *Cuterebra*); hypersensitivity (flea allergy dermatitis, atopy, food allergy); eosinophilic infiltrative disease (eosinophilic granuloma complex, feline bronchial asthma, eosinophilic gastroenteritis/colitis, pulmonary infiltrates with eosinophils [dogs], hypereosinophilic syndrome); infectious diseases (toxoplasmosis, suppurative processes); neoplasia (eosinophilic leukemia, mast cell neoplasia, lymphoma, myeloproliferative disorders, solid tumors), hypoadrenocorticism, pregnancy

Decreased (eosinopenia) in: stress, hyperadrenocorticism, glucocorticoid therapy

Erythrocyte Count (Red Blood Cell [RBC] Count)

Normal range:
Feline: 5.92-9.93 $10^6/\mu L$
Canine: 4.8-9.3 $10^6/\mu L$

Elevated in: dehydration, splenic contraction, polycythemia

Decreased in:
Regenerative anemias
    Acute and chronic hemorrhage
        Gastrointestinal hemorrhage
            Ulcer disease
            Neoplasia
        Trauma
        Coagulopathies
        Ectoparasites (fleas, ticks)
        Endoparasites (hookworms, coccidia)
        Hematuria
Hemolytic anemia
    Immune mediated
    Cold hemagglutinin disease
    Oxidant injury (onion, kale, phenothiazines, methylene blue)
    Parasitic
        Babesiosis
        Haemobartonella felis (Mycoplasma haemofelis)
    Haemobartonella canis (Mycoplasma haemocanis)
    Cytauxzoon felis
    Infectious
        Leptospirosis
        Escherichia coli
    Microangiopathic
        Dirofilariasis
        Vascular neoplasia
        Vasculitis
        Disseminated intravascular coagulation (DIC)

      Zinc or copper toxicosis
      Hypophosphatemia
      Pyruvate kinase deficiency
      Phosphofructokinase deficiency
Nonregenerative anemias
    Renal failure
    Anemia of chronic disease
        Inflammatory disease
        Infectious disease
        Neoplasia
        Drugs
            Chemotherapeutics
            Chloramphenicol
        Sulfadiazine
        Phenylbutazone
    Iron deficiency
        Chronic blood loss
        Nutritional
    Endocrine disease
        Hypothyroidism
        Hypoadrenocorticism
        Hyperestrogenism
            Diethylstilbestrol
            Estradiol
            Sertoli cell tumor
    Infectious
        Feline leukemia virus (FeLV)
        Feline immunodeficiency virus (FIV)
        Ehrlichiosis
        Feline panleukopenia virus (FPV)
Idiopathic aplastic anemia
Red cell aplasia
Myeloproliferative disease
Myelophthisis
Hypersplenism
Lead poisoning
Leukemias

Folate

Normal range:
Feline: 9.7-21.6 ng/mL
Canine: 7.7-24.4 ng/mL
Usually performed in conjunction with serum cobalamin and
   trypsin-like immunoreactivity

Elevated in: exocrine pancreatic insufficiency, small intestinal bacterial overgrowth, dietary supplementation

Decreased in: small intestinal mucosal disease

Fructosamine

Normal range:
Feline and canine: 175-400 µmol/L
    Single sample test that assays mean blood glucose over the previous 1-3 weeks

Elevated: >500 µmol/L: indicates poor glycemic control (hyperglycemia)

Declining or within normal range: indicates improving or adequate glycemic control

Decreased to below lower end of reference range (<300 µmol/L): suggests that patient has experienced significant periods of hypoglycemia over past 1-3 weeks

Values within normal range with PU/PD and polyphagia: suggestive of Somogyi phenomenon

> Note: *Fructosamine values should not be used to make specific adjustments in insulin dosage.*

Gamma Glutamyltransferase (GGT)

Normal range:
Feline: 1-10 U/L
Canine: 1-12 U/L

Elevated: cholestasis—GGT mirrors alkaline phosphatase (intrahepatic, extrahepatic), drugs (dogs [glucocorticoids]), anticonvulsants (phenobarbital, primidone), hepatocellular disease (generally slight increase)

> Note: *Cats with hepatic lipidosis tend to have normal to mildly elevated GGT but greatly elevated alkaline phosphatase levels.*

Decreased: spurious (e.g., laboratory error, lipemic sample), hemolysis

Globulin

Normal range:
Feline: 2.3-5.3 g/dL
Canine: 1.6-3.6 g/dL

Elevated in: dehydration (albumin and total protein also elevated); infection (polyclonal gammopathy; chronic pyoderma, pyometra, chronic periodontitis, feline infectious peritonitis [FIP], bacterial endocarditis, brucellosis, feline immunodeficiency virus [FIV], feline leukemia virus [FeLV], ehrlichiosis [may cause polyclonal or monoclonal gammopathy], leishmaniasis [may cause polyclonal or monoclonal gammopathy], systemic mycoses, chronic pneumonia, bartonellosis, *Mycoplasma haemofelis* infection, Chagas disease, babesiosis); immune-mediated disease (polyclonal gammopathy); neoplasia (polyclonal gammopathy [necrotic or draining tumors, lymphomas, mast cell tumors]); neoplasia (monoclonal gammopathy [multiple myeloma, chronic lymphocytic leukemia, lymphoma]); cutaneous amyloidosis; "idiopathic" monoclonal gammopathy

Glucose

Normal range:
Feline: 64-170 mg/dL
Canine: 70-138 mg/dL

Elevated (hyperglycemia) in: diabetes mellitus, stress (cats), hyperadrenocorticism, pancreatitis, drugs (glucocorticoids, progestagens, megesterol acetate, thiazide diuretics), parenteral nutrition, dextrose-containing fluids, postprandial, acromegaly (cats), diestrus (bitch), pheochromocytoma (dogs), exocrine pancreatic neoplasia, renal insufficiency, head trauma

Decreased (hypoglycemia) in: hepatic insufficiency (portal caval shunts, chronic fibrosis, cirrhosis); sepsis; prolonged sample storage; iatrogenic (insulin therapy, sulfonylurea therapy); toxicity (ethanol ingestion, ethylene glycol); β-cell tumor (insulinoma); extrapancreatic neoplasia (hepatocellular carcinoma or hepatoma, leiomyosarcoma or leiomyoma, hemangiosarcoma, carcinoma [mammary, salivary, pulmonary], leukemia, plasmacytoma, melanoma); hypoadrenocorticism; hypopituitarism; idiopathic hypoglycemia (neonatal hypoglycemia, juvenile hypoglycemia [toy breeds], hunting dog hypoglycemia); renal failure; exocrine pancreatic neoplasia; glycogen storage diseases; severe polycythemia; prolonged starvation; laboratory error

Glucose Tolerance Test

May be used to differentiate type 1 (insulin-dependent) from type 2 (non–insulin-dependent) diabetes mellitus in cats (all dogs are considered to have type 1); results inconsistent; not usually done

Glycosylated Hemoglobin

Assays measure mean blood glucose over the life span of erythrocytes (3-4 months); in dogs, values between 4% and 6% are associated with adequate glycemic control; used less often than fructosamine.

Heartworm Antibody, Feline

Should be interpreted in conjunction with a feline heartworm antigen test

Should be interpreted in light of clinical, clinicopathologic, and radiographic signs

A negative test suggests no exposure to *Dirofilaria immitis* and helps to rule out.

A positive test supports prior exposure but does not confirm active infection.

Heartworm Antigen, Canine

A negative test implies no infection.

A positive test supports active infection.

A sample hemolysis may cause a false-positive result.

A low worm burden may cause a false-negative result.

The result may remain positive for up to 16 weeks after successful adulticide therapy.

Heartworm Antigen, Feline

Should be interpreted in conjunction with a feline heartworm antibody test

Negative test is not useful; may still be positive

Positive test is highly specific; infection is likely

Should be interpreted in light of clinical, clinicopathologic, and radiographic signs

Sample hemolysis may cause false-positive result

Low worm burden or male unisex infection will cause false-negative result

Hematocrit (Packed Cell Volume, PCV)

Normal range:
Feline: 29-48%
Canine: 36-60%

Increased in: dehydration (total protein also increased), polycythemia, splenic contracture

Decreased in: anemia (for more detailed list, see Erythrocyte Count); color of plasma in spun-down hematocrit tube can help determine if icterus (yellow) or intravascular hemolysis (red) is present; buffy coat: may see microfilaria if patient has heartworm disease; mast cells in systemic mastocytosis

Hemoglobin

Hemoglobin concentrations are usually proportional to hematocrit except in rare cases where hemoglobin synthesis defects stimulate polycythemia.

Hemolysis, Prevention in Laboratory Samples

Steps to Prevent Hemolysis:

Fasted patient: Lipemia increases red cell fragility.

Minimize negative pressure (may cause vein to flutter against needle, crushing red cells).

Reposition needle deeper, or slightly rotate to move bevel of needle away from vessel wall.

Resist tendency to increase vacuum by using more negative force; "milk" the vein.

Use vacuum tubes and needles instead of syringes.

Remove needle and specimen tube stopper, and transfer sample directly into open tube.

Aspirate small amount of air from tube to reestablish negative pressure to prevent tops from coming off in transit.

Immunoassays

Assays That Detect all Immunoglobulins to a Specific Antigen in a Serum Sample

Complement fixation

Hemagglutination inhibition

Serum neutralization

Agglutination assay

Agar gel immunodiffusion

Indirect fluorescent antibody

Assays That May Be Used to Detect Specific Immunoglobulins (IgG, IgM, IgA) to Antigens in a Serum Sample

Enzyme-linked immunosorbent assay (ELISA)

Western blot immunoassay

IgM usually first immunoglobulin produced; may indicate recent infection and more likely to be active infection rather than just previous exposure.

Production of immunoglobulin shifts to IgG and/or IgA in days to weeks; indicates more chronic infection and possibly exposure without active disease.

Demonstrating a rising titer with paired samples may be necessary to document active infection.

Insulin

Normal range:
Feline and canine: 15-35 µIU/mL

Elevated: normal or elevated insulin concentration in the presence of hypoglycemia is supportive of insulinoma.

Decreased: decreased insulin levels are not a reliable indicator of diabetes mellitus. Patients with insulin-dependent diabetes mellitus (IDDM) should have low insulin and high glucose levels. Insulin levels in non–insulin-dependent diabetes mellitus (NIDDM) are variable.

Iron-Binding Capacity (Total, TIBC)/Ferritin

Decreased TIBC and decreased ferritin: chronic (not acute) blood loss (intestinal ulceration, hookworm anemia, bleeding from neoplasia, etc.)

TIBC normal to increased, ferritin decreased: iron deficiency

TIBC normal to low, ferritin normal to high: anemia of chronic inflammatory disease

Joint Fluid (Arthrocentesis)

Gross appearance: Evaluate for turbidity (cloudiness), viscosity (does it form a long string when allowed to drip from a needle?), and color (clear, red or hemorrhagic, yellow); yellow color (xanthochromia) may indicate previous hemorrhage, degenerative, traumatic, or inflammatory disease.

Gross appearance, microscopic examination/cytologic evaluation:

Normal
Straw-colored, clear, viscous, firm mucin clot test
1-3 mononuclear cells per high-power field (hpf)
Large and small mononuclear cells with numerous vacuoles and granules; less than 10% are neutrophils (<1 neutrophil/500 erythrocytes if blood contamination has occurred).

Abnormal
Hemarthrosis
Bloody or xanthro-chromic, turbid, reduced viscosity, normal to slightly firable mucin clot test
Hemosiderin-laden macrophage, erythrophagia, moderate neutrophils

Chronic degenerative joint disease
Light yellow, clear to slightly turbid, viscous, normal firm mucin clot
0-20% neutrophils, few to moderate lymphocytes and macrophages

Immune-mediated joint disease (nonerosive)
Yellow to blood-tinged, slight to moderate turbidity, reduced viscosity, friable mucin clot test
15-95% neutrophils, few to moderate lymphocytes, synoviocytes, macrophages

Traumatic
Straw-colored to blood-tinged, slight to moderate turbidity, normal to slightly turbid, normal to slightly friable mucin clot test
Variable neutrophils
May see hemorrhage

Septic
Yellow to blood-tinged to bloody, turbid to purulent, reduced viscosity, friable mucin clot test
90-99% neutrophils
May see microorganisms within cells
Toxic changes in neutrophils

Rheumatoid arthritis (erosive)
Yellow to blood-tinged, turbid, reduced viscosity, friable mucin clot test
20-80% neutrophils
Systemic lupus erythematosus (SLE)–induced polyarthritis: may see LE cells

Lipase

Normal range:
Feline: 10-450 U/L
Canine: 77-695 U/L

Elevated in: most often seen with acute pancreatitis, pancreatic necrosis, pancreatic neoplasia, enteritis, renal disease, glucocorticoids; rarely elevated with certain neoplasms in the absence of pancreatitis.

Note: *Not very sensitive or specific for pancreatic disease*

Lymphocyte Count

Normal range:
Feline: 1200-8000 cells/μL
Canine: 690-4500 cells/μL

Elevated (lymphocytosis): physiologic or epinephrine induced, postvaccination, leukemia (lymphocytic, lymphoblastic), chronic antigenic stimulation (e.g., chronic infection, viremia, immune-mediated, inflammatory bowel disease, cholangiohepatitis, ehrlichiosis, Chagas disease, babesiosis, leishmaniasis, hypoadrenocorticism)

Decreased (lymphopenia): corticosteroid or stress induced; chemotherapy; immunodeficiency (feline leukemia virus [FeLV], feline immunodeficiency virus [FIV]); loss of lymph (chylothorax, lymphangiectasia); viral disease (FeLV/FIV, feline infectious peritonitis [FIP], parvovirus, canine distemper, canine infectious hepatitis)

Magnesium (Mg)

Normal range:
Feline: 1.1-2.3 mEq/L
Canine: 1.2-1.9 mEq/L

Increased in: renal failure or insufficiency, excessive oral intake (antacids, laxatives), excessive parenteral administration

Decreased: dietary, gastrointestinal (malabsorption, chronic diarrhea, pancreatitis, cholestatic liver disease), renal (glomerular disease, tubular disease, postobstructive diuresis, prolonged intravenous fluids, diuretics, digitalis administration, hypercalcemia, hypokalemia), endocrine (diabetic ketoacidosis, hyperthyroidism, primary hyperparathyroidism, primary hyperaldosteronism), multiple endocrine disorders, sepsis, blood transfusion, parenteral nutrition, hypothermia, dialysis, drugs (diuretics, amphotericin B, insulin, glucose, amino acids)

Mean Corpuscular Volume (MCV)

Normal range:
Feline: 37-61 fL
Canine: 58-79 fL

Elevated (macrocytosis) in: regeneration, feline leukemia, feline immunodeficiency virus (FIV), breed-related characteristics (poodles), dyserythropoiesis (bone marrow disease), sample artifact (swelling of RBCs secondary to prolonged storage in EDTA tubes)

Decreased (microcytosis) in: iron deficiency, portosystemic shunt, polycythemia, breed-related characteristics (Akita, Shar-Pei, Shiba Inu)

Methemoglobinemia

Methemoglobin is the form of hemoglobin in which the heme iron has been oxidized from ferrous (Fe^{2+}) to ferric (Fe^{3+}) and is rendered unable to bind and transport oxygen.

Methemoglobinemia is seen in oxidative damage-induced hemolytic anemias and with rare inherited erythrocyte disorders.

Methods of Sample Collection for Cytology

Fine-Needle Biopsy (Aspiration or Nonaspiration Method)

- Surface masses
- Internal masses
- Lymph nodes
- Internal organs
- Fluid collection

Impression Smear

- Exudative cutaneous lesions
- Preparation of cytology samples from biopsy specimens

Scraping

- Flat cutaneous lesions not amenable to fine-needle biopsy
- Preparation of cytologic samples from poorly exfoliative biopsy specimens

Swab

- Vaginal smears
- Fistulous tracts
- Otic swabs
- Nasal, conjunctival swabs

Monocyte Count

Normal range:
Feline: 0-600 cells/µL
Canine: 0-840 cells/µL

Elevated (monocytosis) in: infection (pyometra, abscess, peritonitis, pyothorax, osteomyelitis, prostatitis, *Mycoplasma haemofelis*, blastomycosis, histoplasmosis, *Cryptococcus, Coccidioides*, heartworm disease, other bacteria [e.g., nocardiosis, actinomycosis, mycobacteriosis]); stress or corticosteroid induced; immune-mediated disease (hemolytic anemia, dermatitis, polyarthritis); trauma with severe crushing injury; hemorrhage into tissues or body cavities; neoplasia (tumor necrosis, lymphoma, myelodysplastic disorders, leukemias, myelomonocytic leukemia, monocytic leukemia, myelogenous leukemia)

Myoglobinuria

Brown to dark-red urine with an absence of red blood cells (RBCs) in urine sediment and a positive test for occult blood; seen with generalized muscle disease

Neutrophil Count

Normal range:
Feline: 2500-8500 cells/µL
Canine: 2060-10600 cells/µL

Elevated (neutrophilia): increased production (infection [bacterial, systemic mycoses, protozoal], inflammation [immune-mediated disease, neoplasia, tissue trauma, tissue necrosis]); demargination (stress, hyperadrenocorticism, glucocorticoids); metabolic (uremia, diabetic ketoacidosis); associated with regenerative anemia (hemolytic anemia, hemorrhagic anemia); chronic granulocytic leukemia

Decreased (neutropenia): decreased production (myelophthisis [myeloproliferative disease, lymphoproliferative disease, metastatic neoplasia], myelofibrosis, drug induced [chemotherapeutics, griseofulvin, chloramphenicol, trimethoprim-sulfa, azathioprine, estrogen, phenylbutazone, phenobarbital], infectious [parvovirus, ehrlichiosis, FIV, FeLV {aplastic anemia, myelodysplasia, panleukopenia-like syndrome}]), hypersplenism, idiopathic hypoplasia/aplasia [cyclic neutropenia, immune mediated]); increased consumption (bacteremia/septicemia, severe systemic infection, endotoxemia); hypoadrenocorticism; margination

Osmolality

Plasma osmolality is expected to be decreased in primary polydipsia (psychogenic polydipsia); diabetic ketoacidosis; azotemia; hypernatremia; hyperglycemia; and intoxication with ethylene glycol, ethanol, or methanol.

Plasma osmolality is expected to be increased in primary
polyuria (diabetes insipidus, DI).

There may be considerable overlap in values of primary
polyuria and polydipsia. However, osmolality of less
than 280 mOsm/kg suggests psychogenic polydipsia,
whereas osmolality of greater than 280 mOsm/kg
suggests central DI, nephrogenic DI, or psychogenic
polydipsia.

Packed Cell Volume

See **Hematocrit.**

Parathyroid Hormone (PTH)/Ionized Calcium

Normal range:

PTH:
Feline: 0.0-40.0 pg/mL
Canine: 20.0-130.0 pg/mL

Ionized Calcium:
Feline: 1.16-1.34 mmol/L
Canine: 1.24-1.43 mmol/L

Elevated in: primary hyperparathyroidism (elevated ionized
calcium and mid- to high-elevated PTH), renal or nutritional
secondary hyperparathyroidism (normal or decreased ionized
calcium and elevated PTH), hypercalcemia of malignancy, vitamin D toxicity, granulomatous inflammatory disease

Decreased in: primary hypoparathyroidism (decreased ionized
calcium and low or low-normal PTH)

Phosphorus (P)

Normal range:
Feline: 2.4-8.2 mg/dL
Canine: 2.5-6.0 mg/dL

Elevated in: young, growing animal (also see elevated alkaline
phosphatase); reduced glomerular filtration rate (GFR, acute
renal failure, chronic renal failure); postrenal obstruction, primary hypoparathyroidism, nutritional secondary hyperparathyroidism, hyperthyroidism, acromegaly, hemolysis, intoxication
(hypervitaminosis D, jasmine ingestion); hypoparathyroidism;
dietary excess; metabolic acidosis; iatrogenic (phosphate enemas,

parenteral administration); osteolysis; osteolytic neoplasia; rhabdomyolysis; tumor cell lysis syndrome; sample hemolysis/delayed serum separation

Decreased in: primary hyperparathyroidism (also see increased calcium); nutritional secondary hyperparathyroidism; renal tubular acidosis; vomiting/diarrhea; neoplasia (PTH-like hormone, C-cell thyroid tumors); insulin therapy; diabetic ketoacidosis; Fanconi syndrome; dietary deficiency; decrease intestinal absorption; eclampsia; hyperadrenocorticism; vitamin D deficiency; hyperaldosteronism; aggressive fluid therapy; bicarbonate administration; respiratory or metabolic acidosis

Platelet Count

Normal range:
Feline: 200-500 $10^3/\mu L$
Canine: 170-400 $10^3/\mu L$

Elevated in: essential thrombocytosis, rebound thrombocytosis, polycythemia vera

Decreased (see p. 160): decreased production (infectious [retroviruses: feline immunodeficiency virus, feline leukemia virus; *Ehrlichia*]); increased destruction (immune-mediated thrombocytopenia); sequestration (hypersplenism); increased consumption (hemorrhage, disseminated intravascular coagulation); breed idiosyncrasy (King Charles Spaniels [macrothrombocytes], Greyhounds)

Polymerase Chain Reaction

- PCR amplifies small quantities of DNA to detectable levels.
- Can also be used to detect RNA with a reverse transcriptase step (RT-PCR)
- In general PCR is more sensitive than cytologic, serologic, or histopathologic techniques and is comparable to culture.
- PCR is of great benefit for demonstration of infectious agents, especially if the organism is difficult to culture or cannot be cultured.
- Specificity can be quite high depending on the primers used in the reaction. For example, primers can be designed to detect one bacterial genus but not others. Primers can also be designed to identify one species (e.g., all *Ehrlichia* spp. or only *E. canis*).
- False-positive if sample is contaminated during collection or in laboratory.
- False-negative if sample is handled inappropriately.

Potassium (K)

Normal range:
Feline: 3.4-5.6 g/dL
Canine: 3.6-5.5 g/dL

Elevated in: renal failure (distal renal tubular acidosis, oliguric/anuric); postrenal (obstruction, ruptured bladder); hypoadrenocorticism; acidosis (diabetic ketoacidosis); gastrointestinal (trichuriasis, salmonellosis, perforated duodenal ulcer); chylothorax with repeated pleural fluid drainage; massive muscle trauma; postischemic reperfusion; dehydration; hypoaldosteronism; drugs (potassium-sparing diuretics, ACE inhibitors, propranolol); thrombocytosis; severe leucocytosis (>100,000/µl, hemolysis in breed with high RBC potassium concentration (Akita, English Springer Spaniel, neonates, individuals); hyperkalemic periodic paralysis

Decreased in: alkalosis; dietary deficiency (feline); potassium-free fluids; bicarbonate administration; drugs (penicillins, amphotericin B, loop diuretics, thiazide diuretics); gastrointestinal fluid loss (vomiting and diarrhea, potassium rich); hyperadrenocorticism; hyperaldosteronism; insulin therapy; diuresis caused by diabetic ketoacidosis; renal (postobstructive diuresis, renal tubular acidosis, dialysis); hypokalemic periodic paralysis (Burmese cat, Pit Bull Terrier); renal failure (chronic polyuria); total parenteral nutrition; hypokalemic periodic paralysis (Burmese cats)

Protein, Total (TP)

Normal range:
Feline: 5.2-8.8 g/dL
Canine: 5.0-7.4 g/dL

Elevated in: dehydration (albumin and globulin increased); hyperglobulinemia (chronic inflammation, infection, neoplasia [e.g., multiple myeloma]); spurious (hemolysis, lipemia)

Decreased in: hemorrhage, hypoalbuminemia, liver failure, external plasma loss, gastrointestinal fluid loss, malassimilation, starvation, overhydration, glomerular loss, tumor cachexia

Prothrombin Time (PT)

Normal range:
Feline: 6-11 seconds
Canine: 6-12 seconds
Determines abnormalities in the extrinsic coagulation pathway

Prolonged with deficiencies of factors II, VII, and X

Becomes prolonged before any changes seen in activated coagulation time (ACT) or activated partial thromboplastin time (APTT)

Prolonged with DIC, acquired vitamin K deficiency (rodenticide poisoning), bile insufficiency, and liver failure

Red Blood Cell (RBC) Count

See **Erythrocyte Count.**

Reticulocyte Count

Elevated reticulocyte count is the best indicator of effective erythropoiesis.

Step 1: Multiply percent reticulocytes by red cell count to determine absolute quantity.

Step 2: Correct for reduced red cell mass; multiply absolute reticulocytes by patient's hematocrit divided by mean species hematocrit to obtain the number of reticulocytes per milliliter.

Step 3: Correct for the effect of erythropoietin on the bone marrow reticulocyte release; divide the number of reticulocytes per milliliter by average number of days that a reticulocyte circulates in peripheral blood at that patient's hematocrit to obtain a corrected absolute reticulocyte count.

A corrected absolute reticulocyte count of less than 105,000/mL is indicative of a nonregenerative anemia, whereas strongly regenerative anemias will have a reticulocyte count of greater than 150,000/mL.

Sodium (Na)

Normal range:
Feline: 145-158 mEq/L
Canine: 139-154 mEq/L

Elevated in: dehydration; renal failure; gastrointestinal (GI) fluid loss (Na^+ poor) (vomiting, diarrhea); insensible fluid loss (panting, high ambient temperature, fever); third space loss (i.e., pancreatitis, peritonitis); cutaneous loss (e.g., burns); decreased water intake (limited access to water, primary adipsia); hyperaldosteronemia; increased salt intake (oral, intravenous); spurious (evaporation of serum sample)

Decreased in: hypoadrenocorticism; GI fluid loss (Na^+ rich) (vomiting, diarrhea); severe liver disease; hookworms; renal failure (polyuric); nephrotic syndrome causing effusion; chronic effusions; diuretics; hypotonic fluids; diabetes mellitus; mannitol infusion; burns; excess antidiuretic hormone (ADH); diet (severe sodium restriction); antidiuretic drugs (e.g., vincristine, cyclophosphamide, NSAIDs); myxedema coma of hypothyroidism; psychogenic polydipsia; spurious (hyperlipidemia, marked hyperproteinemia)

Thoracocentesis Fluid

Pyothorax (septic)
Extremely high nucleated cell counts (>50,000/μl), protein
> 3.0 g/dL
Primarily degenerate neutrophils and macrophages
Bacteria seen in white blood cells (WBCs)
Penetrating wounds, foreign body (grass awns), extension of
    bacterial pneumonia or discospondylitis, postoperative
    infection

Nonseptic
Moderate nucleated cell counts (>5000/μl)
Neutrophils, macrophages, eosinophils, lymphocytes
Feline infectious peritonitis (FIP), neoplasia, diaphragmatic
    hernia, lung lobe torsion

Chylous Effusion
Low to moderate nucleated cell counts (400-10,000/μl)
Predominant cell type is small lymphocyte; also neutrophils
    and macrophages
Triglyceride concentration of pleural fluid is greater than that
    of serum.
Idiopathic
Congenital
Secondary to neoplasia, trauma, cardiac disease, fungal
    granuloma, pericardial disease, dirofilariasis, lung lobe
    torsion, diaphragmatic hernia, pericardial diaphragmatic
    hernia, vena caval thrombosis

Hemorrhagic Effusion
Trauma
Coagulopathy
Neoplasia
Lung lobe torsion
Rupture of vessels associated with parasitic infection (Spirocerca
    lupi, Dirofilaria immitis)

Transudates and Modified Transudates
Protein concentrations less than 2.5-3.0 g/dL

Low nucleated cell count (<500-1000/µL)

Macrophages, lymphocytes, mesothelial cells

Right-sided heart failure, pericardial disease, hypoalbuminemia, neoplasia, diaphragmatic hernia

> Note: Neoplastic cells may or may not be present in effusions caused by neoplastic processes.

Eosinophilic Effusion

>10% of leukocytes are eosinophils.

Reported in dogs in association with heartworm disease, systemic mastocytosis, interstitial pneumonia, and disseminated eosinophilic granulomatosis

Thrombocyte Count

See **Platelet Count.**

Thyroid Function Tests

Total T_4 (thyroxine, tetraiodothyronine):

Measures free T4 and protein-bound T4.

Below-normal values suggest hypothyroidism (dogs).

Above-normal values in cats are likely caused by hyperthyroidism.

Below-normal values are also seen with underlying illness (sick, euthyroid).

Free T_4 (FT_4):

Below-normal values suggest hypothyroidism (dogs).

Above-normal values in cats are likely caused by hyperthyroidism.

Not as affected by the suppressive effects of concurrent illness as total T4.

Modified equilibrium dialysis assay is not affected by circulating antithyroid hormone antibodies and therefore is the preferred assay for fT4.

Thyroid-stimulating hormone (TSH) concentration:

Must be interpreted in conjunction with serum T4 and fT4.

Low value for serum T4 and fT4 with a high TSH supports diagnosis of hypothyroidism.

Normal T4 and fT4 and normal TSH rule out hypothyroidism.

TSH and thyroid-releasing hormone (TRH) stimulation tests:

Used to differentiate hypothyroidism from euthyroid sick syndrome.

These tests are not typically done because of availability and
expense of reagents.

T_3 (3,5,3'-triiodothyronine) concentration:
Poor indicator of thyroid function in dogs and cats; not
recommended.

Tests for lymphocytic thyroiditis:
Autoantibodies to circulating thyroid hormone (T4 and T3) and
thyroglobulin (Tg) correlate with lymphocytic thyroiditis.
Tg autoantibodies may be present when T4 and T3 are not;
therefore testing for Tg autoantibodies is considered the
better screening test.
Provides no information about the severity of disease or the
extent of thyroid gland involvement
Hypothyroid dogs may be negative, and euthyroid dogs may
have Tg autoantibodies.
May be used as a prebreeding screening test in breeding dogs

T_3 suppression test:
Administration of T3 to normal cats should suppress pituitary
TSH secretion, decreasing the serum T4 concentration.
Administration of T3 to hyperthyroid cats should have no
suppressive effect.
Confirms hyperthyroidism in cats with occult disease

Toxoplasmosis Antibody Titer

Positive titer indicates exposure but not necessarily active
infection.
Positive IgM titer greater than 1:256 is consistent with active
infection, especially with typical clinical signs.
Fourfold rise in IgG titer of paired samples 2 to 3 weeks apart
also supports active infection.

Triglycerides

Normal range:
Feline: 25-160 mg/dL
Canine: 29-291 mg/dL

Elevated in: postprandial, familial triglyceridemia (Miniature
Schnauzer, other breeds); hyperchylomicronemia of cats (also
observed in dogs); lipoprotein lipase deficiency (cat); endocrine
disorders (hypothyroidism, hyperadrenocorticism, diabetes mellitus); nephrotic syndrome; pancreatitis; cholestasis; drugs (glucocorticoids, megestrol acetate)

Decreased in: not clearly associated with any disease; severe malabsorptive protein-losing enteropathy, hyperthyroidism

Trypsinogen-Like Immunoreactivity (TLI)/ Pancreatic Lipase Immunoreactivity (PLI)

Normal range:

TLI:
Feline: 12.0-82.0 µg/L
Canine: 5.7-45.2.0 µg/L

PLI:
Feline: 0.1-3.5 µg/L
Canine: 0-200 µg/L

Low TLI values (<2.5 µg/L for dogs and <8.0 µg/L for cats) are diagnostic for exocrine pancreatic insufficiency; values between 2.5 and 5.0 µg/L for dogs and 8.0 and 12.0 µg/L for cats are considered equivocal, and the assay should be repeated in 1 month.

High values for TLI are supportive of a diagnosis of acute or chronic pancreatitis.

Elevated values for PLI (>12 µg/L for cats and > 400 µg/L for dogs) are consistent with a diagnosis of pancreatitis.

Patients must be fasted at least 12 hours.

> Note: *These tests are species specific, and samples must be labeled "dog" or "cat" so that the test can be performed correctly.*

Urinalysis

Appearance

Color
Yellow (normal): may be dark amber when concentrated and pale to colorless when diluted. However, color does not always correlate with concentration.
Red or reddish-brown: hematuria, hemoglobinuria, myoglobinuria
Dark brown or black: methemoglobinuria
Yellow-brown to yellow-green: concentrated sample, bilirubinuria, Pseudomonas infection
Orange: bilirubinuria

Turbidity
Normally clear; cloudy urine may contain cellular material, crystals, lipid, and mucus.

Odor
Excess ammonia odor may be detectable in urine infected with urease-producing bacteria.

Specific Gravity

Normal
Feline: 1.025-1.060
Canine: 1.020-1.050

Isosthenuria (1.008-1.012)
Renal failure
Rare cases of polydipsia

Hyposthenuria (<1.008)
Polydipsia/polyuria (e.g., hyperthyroidism, hypercalcemia, hypokalemia, hepatic failure, psychogenic)
Diabetes insipidus

Chemical Properties

pH

Normal: 5.5-7.5 (feline and canine)
Causes of acidic urine: meat-based diet; administration of acidifying agents (e.g., D,L-methionine, NH_4Cl); metabolic acidosis; respiratory acidosis; protein catabolic states; severe vomiting with chloride depletion
Causes of alkaline urine: vegetable-based diet; administration of alkalinizing agents (e.g., $NaHCO_3$, citrate); urinary tract infection by urease-producing bacteria; postprandial alkaline tide; metabolic alkalosis; respiratory alkalosis; renal tubular acidosis (distal tubule)

Protein

Normal: 0-30 mg/dL
Must be interpreted in light of urine specific gravity
Commonly used dipsticks are more sensitive to albumin than globulin.
Increased with glomerular or inflammatory disease

Glucose
Appears in urine if the renal threshold is exceeded
Diabetes mellitus, stress (especially in cats, infuse of dextrose-containing fluids, pheochromocytoma, proximal renal tubular diseases (aminoglycoside toxicity, acute renal failure, Fanconi syndrome, primary renal glucosuria)

Ketones
Test pad measures acetoacetate and acetone but not beta-
hydroxybutyrate, which is responsible for acidosis

Elevated in: diabetes ketoacidosis, starvation, prolonged fasting,
glycogen storage disease, low-carbohydrate diet, persistent fever,
persistent hypoglycemia

Occult Blood
Does not differentiate among erythrocytes (RBCs), hemoglobin,
and myoglobin
Always interpreted in light of urine sediment (evaluation for RBCs)
Erythrocytes—hematuria
Hemoglobin—hemolysis
Myoglobin—rhabdomyolysis

Bilirubin
Detectable in urine before it is elevated in serum
May be found in trace amounts in concentrated samples,
especially in intact males
Bilirubinuria seen in hemolysis, liver disease, extrahepatic
obstruction, fever, starvation

Urobilinogen
Presence indicates normal enterohepatic bilirubin circulation.

Urinary Sediment Examination

Red Blood Cells (RBCs)
Normally, zero to occasional RBCs; excessive RBCs termed
hematuria (see p. 34)

White Blood Cells (WBCs)
Normally, zero to occasional WBCs
Excessive WBCs termed *pyuria;* indicates urinary tract infection
but does not localize the site of infection

Epithelial Cells
Squamous and transitional cells, little diagnostic significance
Increased transitional cells may be seen with infection,
neoplasia, and irritation of the urinary tract.

Casts
Cylindrical molds of renal tubules composed of aggregated
proteins or cells that localize disease to the kidney
Occasional hyaline or granular cast may be normal; cellular
casts are always abnormal.

Hyaline casts: protein precipitates (Tamm-Horsfall mucoprotein and albumin); seen with proteinuric renal disease (glomerulonephritis, amyloidosis), small numbers with fever and exercise

Granular casts: degeneration of cells in casts or precipitation of filtered plasma proteins; suggest ischemic or nephrotoxic renal tubular injury

Cellular casts: WBC casts (pyelonephritis), RBC casts (fragile, rare in dogs and cats), renal epithelial cell casts (acute tubular necrosis or pyelonephritis)

Fatty casts: lipid granules (nephrotic syndrome or diabetes mellitus)

Waxy casts: final stage of degeneration of granular casts (suggest intrarenal stasis)

Organisms: Small numbers of bacteria may contaminate voided or catheterized samples but usually not enough to be seen in urine sediment unless sample is allowed to incubate. Presence of large numbers of bacteria in sediment suggests urinary tract infection. Yeast and fungal hyphae usually are contaminants.

Crystals
Usually of little diagnostic value; typically found in normal urine
Acidic urine may contain urate, calcium oxalate, and cystine crystals.
Alkaline urine may contain struvite, calcium phosphate, calcium carbonate, amorphous phosphate, and ammonium biurate crystals.
Bilirubin crystals may be seen with concentrated samples or with bilirubinuria.
Urate crystals may be seen in Dalmatians and with liver disease or portosystemic shunts.
Struvite crystals are seen in cats with idiopathic lower urinary tract disease, dogs, and cats with struvite urolithiasis.
Calcium oxalate in oliguric acute renal failure (ARF) suggests ethylene glycol intoxication.
Cystine crystals, when abnormal, suggest cystinuria.

Other Findings in Sediment
Sperm in intact male dogs
Parasite ova; *Dioctophyma renale, Capillaria plica*
Microfilariae
Lipid droplets (diabetes mellitus, nephrotic syndrome, in cats with degeneration of lipid-laden tubular cells)

Common Bacteria Seen in Urinary Tract Infections
Escherichia coli
Proteus spp.
Staphylococcus spp.
Pasteurella multocida
Enterobacter spp.
Klebsiella spp.
Pseudomonas aeruginosa

Urine Cortisol/Creatinine Ratio

Very sensitive, but not very specific test for
hyperadrenocorticism
Good test to rule out hyperadrenocorticism but not to diagnose

Urine Protein/Creatinine Ratio

More accurate than dipstick protein estimation
Normal values: dogs less than 0.3, cats less than 0.6

von Willebrand Factor

Variable degrees of expression of factor for von Willebrand disease
(vWD), a common, inherited hemostatic disorder (rare in cats)
Dogs with levels less than 30% are prone to spontaneous
bleeding (e.g., epistaxis).
Classification of vWD in dogs:
Type I: low concentration of normal von Willebrand factor
Type II: low-normal concentration of abnormal von
Willebrand factor
Type III: absence of von Willebrand factor
Hemostatic screening tests usually are normal in dogs with vWD.
Buccal mucosal bleeding time is the exception—best screening test.

White Blood Cell (WBC) Count

Normal range:
Feline: 3.5-16.0 10^3/μL
Canine: 4.0-15.5 10^3/μL

Elevated in: infection (bacterial, systemic mycoses); physiologic
leucocytosis; metabolic (stress, glucocorticoids); inflammation
(immune-mediated disease, neoplasia, tissue trauma, tissue necrosis); leukemia, associated with responsive anemia (hemorrhagic anemia, hemolytic anemia)

Decreased in: decreased production, increased consumption,
neutropenia secondary to phenobarbital administration